A Laboratory Manual of Physical Pharmaceutics

A Laboratory Manual of Physical Pharmaceutics

Sadhan Kumar Dutta

PhD (Pharmacy, J.U.)

Retired Professor of Pharmacy, Department of Pharmaceutical Technology,
Jadavpur University, Kolkata-32
Author of the text book titled "Principles of Physical Pharmacy and Biophysical Chemistry"

and

Kalyan Kumar Sen

M. Pharm., PhD (J.U.)

Principal and Professor in Pharmaceutics
Gupta College of Technological Sciences
Ashram more, G.T.Road, Asansol, W.B.

PharmaMed Press

An imprint of BSP Books Pvt. Ltd.
4-4-309/316, Giriraj Lane,
Sultan Bazar, Hyderabad - 500 095.

A Laboratory Manual of Physical Pharmaceutics
***by* Sadhan Kumar Dutta and Kalyan Kumar Sen**

Fifth Reprint 2024

Published by

PharmaMed Press
An imprint of BSP Books Pvt. Ltd.
4-4-309/316, Giriraj Lane, Sultan Bazar, Hyderabad - 500 095.
Phone: 040-23445688, 23445600; Fax: 91+40-23445611
E-mail: info@pharmamedpress.com
www.pharmamedpress.com/pharmamedpress.net

Printed at

Aditya Offset Process (I) Pvt. Ltd.
Hyderabad.

Price: Rs. 225.00
ISBN: 978-93-87593-82-4 (Paperback)

PREFACE

This book aims to bring together the principles and practical aspects of implementing physicochemical methods and their application in the pharmaceutical technology. The importance of thorough understanding of Physical Principles to the students of pharmaceutical technology, medicine and biochemistry is now well established. The stimulus for the creation of this book was a authors' interest in developing an alternative and lucidly elaborated practical methods of physical pharmaceutics according to students' need. This book illustrates various primary experiments of physical pharmaceutics covering syllabus of PCI and different universities. The authors are grateful to a host of highly talented and widely referred authors of the subjects of earlier years and present days.

Finally the printed version of the book sees the light of the dawn, courtesy PharmaMed Press. Thanks and acknowledgements are due to the publishing house.

It is our fervent hope that this book will provide stimulation, inspiration, and confidence to the students so that they will be do these practical with better understanding and ease. Further suggestions are sought for future guidance.

- Authors

CONTENTS

Preface .... (v)

Experiment - 1

Required for Physical Pharmacy and Pharmaceutics Laboratory **1**

Experiment - 1A

Calibration of a Thermometer 4

Experiment - 1B

Statistical Evaluation of the Data 6

Experiment - 2

Partial Miscibility - Phenol-Water System **7**

Experiment - 2A

Determination of the Percentage of Phenol along the Tie Line (x,y) Drawn at any Temperature in the Phase Diagram Curve: Transition Temperature vs % of Phenol 9

Experiment - 3

Ternary Phase Study **10**

Experiment - 4

Temperature-Composition Curves for a Solid-Solid System **13**

Experiment - 5

Heat of Solution/Heat of Precipitation **15**

Experiment - 6

Determination of Solubility and Heat of Solution **18**

Experiment - 7

Solubility and Qualitative Determination of Solubility Behavior **20**

Experiment – 8

Use of the Dielectric Constant – Solubility Relationship for Blending Pharmaceutical Solvent System 22

Experiment – 9

Measurement of pH and Buffer Solutions 30

Experiment – 10

The Effect of pH on the Solubility of a Slightly Soluble Weak Acid 34

Experiment – 11

Viscosity of Liquids 37

Experiment – 12

Surface and Interfacial Tension Measurement 40

Experiment – 13

Determination of the Critical Micelle Concentration (CMC) of a given Surfactant by Surface Tension Method 49

Experiment – 14

Chemical Kinetics 52

Experiment – 15

Chemical Kinetics Involving Second-order Reactions 56

Experiment – 16

Conductivity of Solutions 58

Experiment – 16A

To Determine the Cell Constant of a Given Conductivity Cell 60

Experiment – 16B

Determination of the Dissociation Constant, K_a of a Weak Acid, (Say Acetic Acid) at Various Dilutions and hence to Verify Ostwald's Dilution Law Conductometrically 61

Experiment - 16C

Determination of the Solubility of a Sparingly Soluble Salt (AgCl) by Conductivity Method at Room Temperature and hence also KS_p (Solubility Product of AgCl) 63

Experiment - 17

Refractometry **64**

Experiment - 17A

Determination of the Concentration of a Supplied Sample (say KCl, NaCl or $BaCl_2$) in Solution by using a Refractometer 65

Experiment - 17B

Determination of the Percent Composition of a Binary Liquid Mixture of Two Liquids using a Refractometer 67

Experiment - 18

Polarimeter **69**

Experiment - 18A

Determination of the Specific Rotation of an Optically Active Substance and hence to verify its Purity and also to Determine the Concentration of the given Substance in Solution 71

Experiment - 18B

Determination of the Composition of a given Binary Mixture of Two Components in which one is Optically Active 73

Experiment - 18C

Determination of the Order of Acid-Hydrolysis of Sucrose (or any other Optically Active Substance) at Room Temperature using a Polarimeter 75

Experiment - 19

Experiment on Partition Co-efficient **77**

Experiment - 19A

Determination of the Partition Coefficient of Benzoic Acid between Water and Benzene 79

Experiment - 19B

Determination of the Distribution Coefficient of Salicylic Acid between Water and Benzene ... 81

Experiment - 19C

Determination of the Partition (Distribution Equilibrium) Constant of Iodine between Water and Carbon Tetrachloride (CCl_4) or Chloroform ($CHCl_3$) ... 83

Experiment - 20

Adsorption at a Solid-liquid Interface ... 85

Experiment - 20A

Determination of the Specific Surface Area (area/g) of a given Powder (Activated Charcoal as an Example) ... 87

Experiment - 20B

Verification of Freundlich's Adsorption Isotherm for the Adsorbate (Oxalic Acid/Acetic Acid/ Benzene Acid) and the Adsorbent (Activated Charcoal/any other Inert Adsorbent of Pharmaceutical Interest ... 90

Experiment - 21

Hydrophile - Lipophile Balance (HLB) ... 91

Experiment - 22

On Colloidal Dispersions ... 94

Experiment - 23

Suspensions ... 97

Experiment - 23A

Sedimentation Rate ... 98

Experiment - 23B

Sedimentation Rate in the Presence of Surfactants and Electrolytes ... 100

Experiment - 23C

Relationship between Suspension Caking and Zeta Potential ... 101

Experiment - 23D

Determination of the Concentration Range which the Electrolyte (say, $AlCl_3$) Acts as a Deflocculating Agent for Kaolin Suspension (say of 10%) 102

Experiment - 24

Surfactants, Emulsions, and Solubilization 104

Experiment - 25

Rheology (I.e. Flow Properties) 110

Experiment - 26

Properties of Solids 112

Experiment - 26A

Determination of the Bulk Density of a given Powdered (or granular) Sample 114

Experiment - 26B

Determination of the True Density of a given Powdered (or granular) Sample 115

Experiment - 27

Particle Size Distribution Techniques 116

Experiment - 27A

Sieve Method 118

Experiment - 27B

Microscopy Method 120

Experiment - 27C

Anderson Pipette Method 122

Experiment - 28

Thixpotropy Measurement 125

Experiment - 29

Measurement of Angle of Repose 127

Experiment - 29A

The Effect of Glidant Concentration on the Angle of Repose of a given Sample 130

Experiment - 30

Determination of Swelling Index and Swelling Rate Constant of a polymer 131

Experiment - 31

Tablet Coating Procedures 133

Experiment - 31A

Sub-coating 134

Experiment - 31B

Sub-coating 138

Experiment - 31C

Coloring 141

Experiment - 32

Evaluation of Tablets 146

Experiment - 33

Thermodynamics of Solubilization (i.e. Micellar Solubilization) 147

Experiment - 33A

Thermodynamics of Micellization 150

Experiment - 1

Required for Physical Pharmacy and Pharmaceutics Laboratory

Required Materials:

1. Texts: Dutta S.K., Principles of Physical Pharmacy and Biophysical Chemistry Martin A.N., Physical Pharmacy
2. Laboratory Notebook – bound and duplicate numbered pages
3. Long white laboratory gowns
4. Set of metric weights
5. Box of cleansing tissues
6. Graph papers

Laboratory Procedure:

1. All experiments will be performed by pairs or 3 in a group. Each student must record data in his or her own Laboratory Notebook and prepare an **individual report** to be submitted.
2. A full comprehension of the assigned work will be expected of each student prior to the actual experimentation. In this manner, a student can plan his or her work for completion within the assigned time-schedule.
3. Students are expected to observe proper laboratory etiquette, conduct and attire.
4. Proper laboratory techniques learned in other courses must be practiced.
5. Many experiments require the use of delicate and expensive equipments and, as such, **special care must be taken** under these circumstances.
6. Laboratory cleanliness in the working areas will be strongly encouraged.
7. Equipment signed out must be returned clean and dry before leaving the laboratory.
8. Students **must check out** with the laboratory instructor before leaving the laboratory.

Laboratory Notebook: The following rules must be adhered to:

1. Each page must be dated.
2. All experimental data must be the **original record**; and not copies of date originally recorded on separate pieces of paper. If some sacrifice of neatness is necessary to adhere to this rule, then it is a worthwhile sacrifice.
3. Besides data, any observations and calculations made should be included in your notebook.
4. A **carbon copy of your data** must be submitted **before leaving** for the day. **No data should be accepted at a later date.**

Laboratory Report:

The laboratory report must be handled in at a previously announced time, generally one week after the experiment had been performed. Failure to submit reports on time will prevent proceeding to the next experiment and also will result in a lower grade for the report.

The report should include:

1. A brief statement as to the purpose of the experiment
2. A description of the experimental procedure, concise enough to be repeated by another person
3. Tabulation of raw data and calculated data.
4. Sample calculations
5. Neatly drawn and labeled graphs
6. Conclusions
7. Literature references.

EQUIPMENT LIST

Name:____________________

Section No.__________ **Desk No.**__________

(For instructor's use)

S. No.	Quantity	Equipment		Size
1	1.	Burette with Teflon plug	-	50 mL
2	1.	Volumetric pipette	-	50 mL
3	2.	Volumetric pipette	-	25 mL
4	1.	Volumetric pipette	-	10 mL
5	2.	Volumetric pipette	-	5 mL
6	2	Volumetric pipette	-	2 mL

Table *Contd...*

S. No.	Quantity	Equipment		Size
7	2	Volumetric pipette	-	1 mL
8	1	Volumetric pipette	-	1 mL
9	1	Graduated pipette	-	10 mL
10	1	Volumetric flask	-	500 mL
11	2	Volumetric flask	-	250 mL
12	2	-do-	-	100 mL
13	2	-do-	-	50 mL
14	1	Erlenmeyer flask	-	500 mL
15	2	-do-	-	250 mL
16	2	-do-	-	100 mL
17	2	-do-	-	50 mL
18	2	Funnel	-	1(medium) + 1 (small)
19		Thermometer	-	
20		Water-bath with rings	-	1 pc
21		Tripod	-	1
22		Bunsen burner with tubing	-	
23		Stirring rods	-	
24		Wash bottle fittings	-	Large + small
25		Spatula, spoon type	-	
26		Weighing bottles	-	
27		Burette clamps	-	

Students should have with them the following items (purchased):

1. Test tube brush (2) Detergent (3) Glass-marking pencil (4) Wire-gauge 6" x 6"

Student's signature (in)

Instructor's signature (in) Date

Student's signature (out)

Instructor's signature (out) Date

Experiment - 1A

Calibration of a Thermometer

1. Since a major portion of the laboratory exercises in this course involves measurement of weight, volume, temperature, concentrations, etc. demonstrations of proper techniques, to be used in **all** laboratories, will be given by the instructor(s). You will be expected to continue to use these techniques throughout the year and subsequent years of your professional career.
2. Thermometer Calibration: The purpose of this experiment is to acquaint the student(s) with the fact that no instrument is absolutely accurate.

   The objective of this experiment is to calibrate a thermometer at two places on its range. This is done using the ice point and boiling point of water, taking into account the necessary corrections.

Procedure:

(a) ***Ice-point determination:*** A 100 mL beaker is filled with chopped ice. The temperature is determined with the thermometer supplied employing good stirring. Several readings are to be taken (and recorded in the notebook) until successive readings are constant. The use of a towel wrapped around the beaker will act as insulation. Does it make a significant difference? If yes, why? Experimental and theoretical ice-points temperatures are then compared.

(b) ***Boiling point determination:*** A wash bottle, made of glass, is modified by removing the delivery tubing (i.e. the longest piece of tubing) and replacing it with the thermometer supplied. The depth of the thermometer is adjusted so as to minimize steam and steam-convection without risking the danger of splashing water on to the thermometer. It is to be ensured that there is an opening to the atmosphere and that boiling chips are used before heating the water.

The temperature read on the thermometer and the temperature of the emergent stem are recorded. After stem corrections the experimental and theoretical boiling points are compared.

Barometric pressure is to be noted and the corrected pressure and the corrected boiling point of water at that pressure are recorded in the notebook.

SUMMARY

The corrections which would be necessary in using the laboratory thermometer are to be recorded and used to get a correct reading.

This process is known as calibration which is required for calibrating each and every equipment such as burette, pipette, weight box, etc. which are required for routine laboratory and research works.

Experiment - 1B

Statistical Evaluation of the Data

The purpose of this experiment is to enable the student to use simple statistical procedures in evaluating the data generated.

Procedure:

Accurately measure 100.00 mL of water (may be with the help a standardized burette or pipette in a 100.00 mL graduate) and the content is transferred carefully into the 250 mL beaker that was supplied, allowing all of the water to drain into the beaker. The meniscus is marked by placing a line-mark with a glass-marking pencil and the beaker is emptied of its contents. The beaker is filled up with water up to its calibration mark and the volume of its contents is measured with the 50 mL graduate (estimated to the nearest 0.5 mL).

The process is repeated ten times.

Calculate the mean, median, mode, standard deviation and standard error of the experiment.

Do your results follow a normal distribution curve?

Experiment - 2

Partial Miscibility – Phenol-Water System

Liquids are often miscible in all proportions but there are a number of pairs in which the solubility of each in the other is limited. Usually both liquids become more soluble as the temperature is increased, and eventually a critical solution temperature is reached above which the liquids are miscible in all proportions.

The temperature-composition curve of such systems when experimentally determined permits a complete understanding of the behavior of any system of two liquids, and the interpretation of the curve constitutes an important exercise in the application of the phase rule.

Phenol and water make a particularly suitable pair because the critical solution temperature (CST) occurs at a convenient temperature, below the boiling point of either component. Phenol is not ordinarily a liquid, but the first portion of water lowers the melting point of the solid below room temperature to produce a liquid-liquid system.

Apparatus:

Beckmann molecular weight apparatus, stirring rod, 2 mL and 10 mL pipette, 0°C-100°C thermometer.

Procedure:

5 g of phenol, weighed out to 0.1 g and 5 mL of water are placed into the inner tube along with the glass stirrer and the thermometer. After inserting it into the air-jacket (in order to reduce the rate of heating and cooling) the entire assembly is placed into a 1 L beaker filled with water. The assembly is now heated to raise the temperature to about 60°C by boiling the water and stirring the mixture. At a certain temperature the turbid mixture will suddenly become clear because at this temperature the phenol and water are miscible. The temperature is recorded to the nearest tenth of a degree. The tube is then, lifted out of the hot water and the solution is allowed to cool while being stirred. The solution becomes milky again and the temperature at which first turbidity appears should be the same as previously recorded. Two or three checks should be made with the rising and falling temperatures. Close agreement will be obtained if the temperature changes slowly.

2 mL of water is added from a pipette and the determinations are repeated. This time the temperature of complete miscibility will be higher.

The determinations are repeated 10 times adding 2 mL of water each time. The experiment is continued until the temperature of complete miscibility has risen passed through a maximum and fallen below 60°C.

Calculations:

The percentage-composition by weight (% w/w) of the different mixtures is to be calculated and then a plot of temperature of complete miscibility versus the corresponding composition is to be obtained. The critical solution temperature (CST) may, then, be determined from the graph. This CST is also known as upper consolute temperature.

The other system that shows lower critical solution temperatures or lower consolute temperature can also be studied. One such example is the water-tri-ethyl amine system exhibiting CST at around 18°C-19°C.

Another type exhibiting both upper and lower critical temperature can also be studied. The most common example is the Nicotine Water system showing CST's of 208°C and 60°C respectively and β-picoline/water system has 153°C/49°C.

Extended Experimentation:

Influence of Foreign substances on CST:

The critical solution temperature is very sensitive to the pressure of any impurity or foreign substance. The CST of phenol-water system would be raised by 20°C if naphthalene be added to make a concentration of only 0.1 M. Again, the consolute temperature (4°C) of the system acetic acid/cyclohexane is raised by about 18°C when 1% water is present in the acetic acid. This fact is utilized in ascertaining the presence and even the amount of impurities present in a sample.

Generally, CST is raised by an impurity if the later is soluble in one of the phases only; the CST is lowered when a third substance present is soluble in both the liquids. The use of soap increases the mutual solubilities of cresols and water and enables us to obtain clear commercial preparations of disinfectant solutions like lysols at ordinary temperature.

Experiment – 2A

Determination of the Percentage of Phenol along the Tie Line (x,y) Drawn at any Temperature in the Phase Diagram Curve: Transition Temperature vs % of Phenol

Materials: Materials and method as in the previous experiment as described; observation as above.

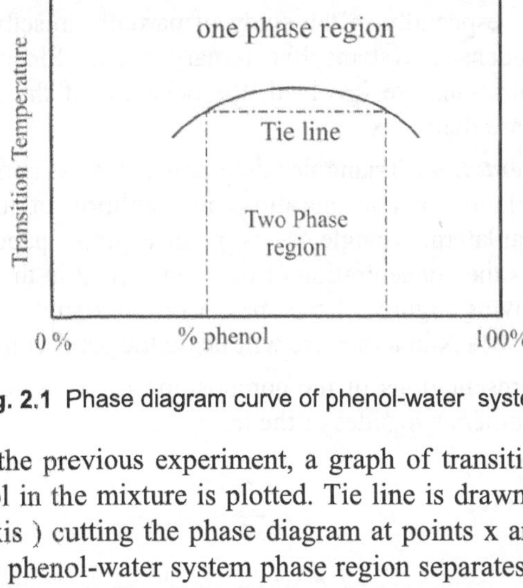

Fig. 2.1 Phase diagram curve of phenol-water system.

Graph: As in the previous experiment, a graph of transition temperature. Vs % of phenol in the mixture is plotted. Tie line is drawn at 50°C (a line parallel to x-axis) cutting the phase diagram at points x and y. Along the tie line, xy, the phenol-water system phase region separates into two layers and % of phenol in the upper layer (x%) as well as in the lower layer (y%) remain the same. These values can be determined by drawing perpendiculars at x and y to the X-axis.

Result: % phenol in the upper layer = x% and % phenol in the lower layer = y% along x-y tie line at the experimental temperature.

Experiment - 3

Ternary Phase Study

In a ternary system if all the three components form a homogeneous single phase, which is the minimum number of phases, the degrees of freedom, F will be maximum, i.e.

$$F = C - P + 2 = 3 - 1 + 2 = 4$$

The four variables to be defined are temperature, total pressure, and concentrations of any two of the components. If the first two are fixed, the equilibria in such systems would be defined by the two concentrations only. Such cases arise especially in the study of partially miscible liquids or in the case of condensed systems like ternary alloys. Since, only the two variable concentrations are involved, the behavior of the systems can be described by phase diagrams.

Graphical Presentation: Triangular diagrams are most commonly used to indicate the variation of concentrations in equilibria of three-component systems. An equilateral triangle is taken on a graph paper each side of which represents the concentration of one component in the mixture. Thus, in the accompanying Figure 3.1 the apex A of the triangle indicates pure A (i.e. 100%) and 50% A in a mixture will lie on the parallel line XX.

Identical representations of the composition of B and C (100%) C are made along the others two sides of the triangle.

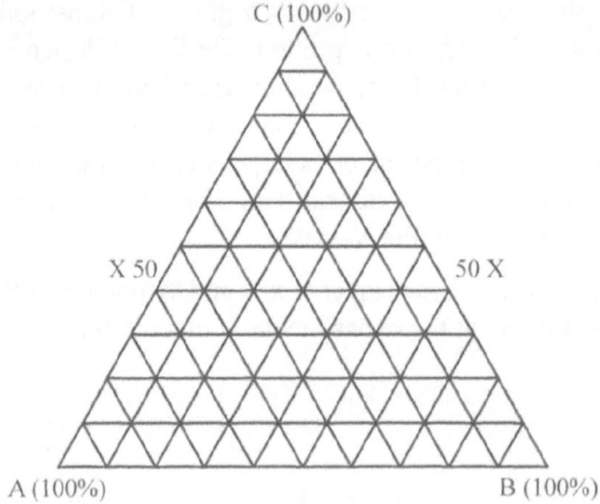

Fig. 3.1 Ternary Phase Diagram.

Example: Water and chloroform are partially miscible and if acetic acid is gradually added a (100%) complete homogeneous mixture is possible. (x) Such systems are chosen for practical purpose.

Procedure:

Chloroform and acetic acid are completely miscible in each other forming a uniformly distributed homogeneous mixture. A series of solutions (say 10) are prepared by varying the concentration of one in another by 10% w/w increment (weight of individual liquid component is calculated by multiplying the volume of the liquid by its respective density component at the temperature of the experiment). The first one is a liquid of 100% pure chloroform and each of the remaining eight is a mixture of chloroform and acetic acid of desired composition. The last container contains only pure acetic acid.

Now the eight mixtures are titrated one by one by adding water from a burette and the end point of each titration is indicated by the appearance of turbidity in each case. The volume of water required for each titration is noted (the density of water may be taken as 1 or it may be determined experimentally at that temperature of the experiment).

Alternatively, we may start by taking mixture of water and chloroform of varying composition. All will become turbid mixtures and in cases where one is added in appreciable amounts so as to exceed the mutual solubility limits, two conjugate solutions will be formed separated into two layers. The turbid solutions are then titrated with the third liquid C, i.e. acetic acid; it would be distributed between the two layers being completely miscible with both the liquids until the end points are obtained indicated by the disappearance of turbidity in each case. The temperature should be kept constant throughout the procedure.

The variation in the miscibility of A and B when increasing amounts of C (the third liquid which is miscible with both) are added is shown as in the figure below (Figure 3.2). If we have a solution mixture of A and B in the proportion as at point Z, then this mixture will separate into two layers of conjugate solutions having composition as at x and y.

As C is gradually added, the composition (overall) of the mixtures of three components will change along AC. For a mixture of composition z_i the system is still hetero- C (CH_3COOH) generous and the two ternary conjugates layers will have concentrations denoted by x_i and y_i. The line x_iy_i passing through z_i is called a tie-line. The tie-line is a mixture of the miscibility gap. As more and more C is added the tie-lines become shorter and shorter till these merge to a K point at K_i. The curve, xk_iky, obtained by joining the terminates of the tie-lines (i.e. the limiting values of the k_i miscibilities of A and B and B in A in presence of C) y_i demarcates the zone of heterogeneous existence of the x_i z_i system. Outside the curve xk_iky

for any compound the ternary system will be homogeneous and inside the (A) system is heterogeneous. The curve xky is called the ($CHCl_3$) x z y H_2O binodal curve. Complete miscibility by merging of two (B) layers would occur only at k, i.e. the composition of the Figure 2 two layers at this point become identical and this point k is called the plait-point of the system. At a given temperature and fixed pressure, the plait-point will have a definite (i.e. fixed) composition which means it is an invariable point at a given temperature, i.e. F=0. With temperature change, the binodal curve and hence the plait-point will also change. Another well-known ternary system of this type is water-alcohol-ether.

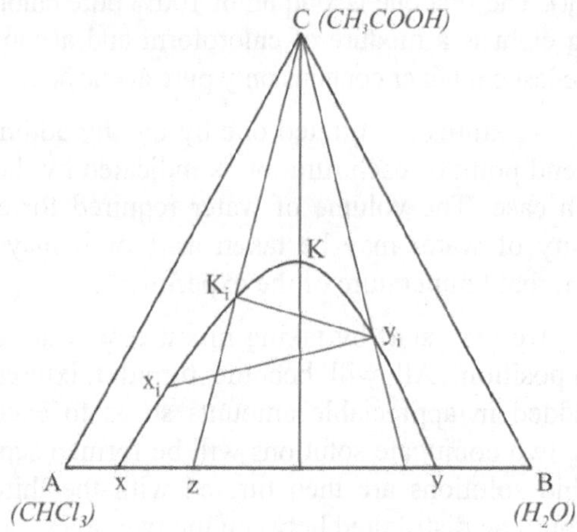

Fig. 3.2 Ternary Phase diagram.

Experiment - 4

Temperature-Composition Curves for a Solid-Solid System

The freezing point or melting point of a pure solid compound is the temperature at which solid crystals are in equilibrium with the liquid phase under its own vapor pressure. If a substance is pure the melting point will be sharp. If a second component is present, depending on the composition, the melting point will be different, generally lower than the melting points of both pure substances.

In pharmaceutical systems, some compounds are known to mutually lower their respective melting point below that of room temperature, yielding a liquid mass without heating; camphor and menthol are excellent examples. Such a phenomenon is known as eutexia, a common incompatibility when dealing with solid mixtures. Actually, eutexia is a more general phenomenon and involves any mutual lowering of melting point whether it be below or above room temperature. The system to be studied here has a eutectic point above room temperature but it serves to illustrate the general procedure required to determine the temperature-composition curve of a binary solid mixture, and especially the eutectic point.

Apparatus:

Beckmann freezing point apparatus 0°C-200°C thermometer.

Procedure:

Samples required for the purpose are

(a) Pure benzoic acid

(b) Mixtures of benzoic acid and cinnamic acid, in mole-percent of 10, 20, 30, 50, 70, 90

(c) Pure cinnamic acid

Approximately 2.5 g of each sample are placed into the inner tube of the freezing point apparatus.

After having heated the tube so as to melt the solid, the tube is placed into the air-jacket and then into the large flask filled with water.

This would ensure a moderate rate of cooling. It is to be ensured that the bulb of the thermometer is completely immersed into the liquid mass. The temperature of the liquid is recorded immediately and then at 15 second intervals and continued until complete solidification is observed or when the temperature drops below 30°C.

Cooling curves are drawn for the various samples, plotting temperature versus time. From these the freezing point of each sample is determined. The freezing temperature-composition diagram is, then, drawn and the various phases labeled indicating the position of eutectic point and hence its value.

Reference: Weissberger, Physical methods of Organic chemistry Vol.1, Part-1.

Remington, Practice of Pharmacy.

Experiment - 5

Heat of Solution/Heat of Precipitation

From thermodynamic considerations it is observed that the heat of solution can be of considerable value in understanding the solution process, particularly the energy changes associated with the dissociation of crystal lattices and ion hydration. This can be seen from the following relationship:

Heat of solution = Crystal lattice energy – Sum of ion hydration energies.

Heats of solution are often difficult to measure directly be calorimetric methods, but for slightly soluble salts, their converse, the heat of precipitation, are easily measured. It may be recalled that the heat of precipitation is just minus the heat of solution.

For example: $Ag^+ + Cl^- = AgCl$; $\Delta H = -15{,}650$ cal $mole^{-1}$

$AgCl \rightleftharpoons Ag^+ + Cl^-$; $\Delta H = +15{,}650$ cal $mole^{-1}$

The heats of precipitation of AgCl, AgBr, and AgI will be measured by using a simply constructed calorimeter and determining the total heat evolved during the reaction.

Procedure:

(a) ***Construction of calorimeter:*** A 250 mL Erlenmeyer flask is placed in 600 mL beaker. Pack the space between the flask and the beaker with glass wool and wrap the beaker with a towel. A thermometer (0.1 interval) is inserted through a rubber stopper that tightly fits the flask. (Use GLOVES WHEN HANDLING THE GLASS WOOL).

(b) ***Heat capacity of the calorimeter:*** 0.25 M HCl is pipetted out and taken into the Erlenmeyer flask. The thermometer is placed in place and the solution temperature is checked at least for two minutes till a constant reading is obtained. From a graduated cylinder 11.0 mL of 2.5 M NaOH solution is added. The thermometer is replaced immediately and temperature readings are taken every 30 seconds and the highest temperature that develops is recorded. The procedure is repeated to get concurrent readings.

(c) ***Heat of precipitation:*** The above procedure is repeated with 100 mL of 0.25 M $AgNO_3$, and 11 mL of 2.5 M NaCl, NaBr, and NaI solutions respectively. For each salt solution duplicate runs should be performed.

(d) Assuming that the heat of neutralization for a strong acid with a strong base, is constant which is – 13,630 calories (approximately) the heat q, in Cal, that would be liberated in the complete reaction of 100 mL of 0.25 M HCl and 11 mL of 2.5 M NaOH, is calculated using the equation :

$$Q = m.s\,(t_2 - t_1) = C_v\,(t_2 - t_1)$$

When C_v is the heat capacity of the calorimeter (taking into account m = mass, and s = specific heat of the assembled calorimeter).

The heat capacity in calories per degree using the data from part B is computed. This is in effect, the heat capacity of the calorimeter plus 111 g of solution.

(e) Using the heat capacity just calculated and the temperature change observed for the various reactions, in part C, q, the amount of heat liberated is calculated in each case. This is then the heat of precipitation.

Remark: Compare the values for AgCl, AgBr and AgI and be prepared to discuss the possible reasons for the differences in ΔH and also account for the differences in the ΔH values for the three silver halides.

To determine the Heat of Ionization of a weak acid (say active acid).

First water-equivalent of the apparatus set-up is to be determined. Let it be ω.

Ionization of acetic acid:

Step 1: $CH_3COOH + H_2O \rightleftharpoons CH_3COO^- + H_3O^+$, ΔH = heat of ionization.

Step 2: Reaction of H_3O^+ with OH^- ions i.e. neutralization process

$$\Delta H = 13.6 \text{ Kcal mole}^{-1}$$
$$= 13600 \text{ cals mole}^{-1}$$

Because, heat of neutralization of a strong acid with a strong base is always constant and it is 13500 cals $mole^{-1}$ ≈ 13600 cals/mole (taken for calculation)

$$\Delta H_{total} = \Delta H_1 + \Delta H_2 \qquad \text{.....(1)}$$

Data: Temperature of 0.5 N acetic acid = t_a = ... °C

Temperature of 0.5 N sodium hydride = t_6 = ... °C

Constant temperature of the mixture = t_m = ... °C

After neutralization,

250 mL of 0.5 N CH_3COOH ≡ 250 mL of 0.5 N NaOH, Let Q be the amount of heat evolved.

$$\Delta H_{total} = \Sigma Q \qquad \text{.....(2)}$$

where Q = Heat of neutralization of 0.5 N CH_3COOH (250 mL) with 0.2 N NaOH (250 mL), and $Q = m_a.S_a.\ \Delta t_a + m_b.S_b.\ \Delta t_m + \omega_a.\ \Delta t_a$

where, m_a = mass of acid = 250 g (density of 0.2 N acid = 1), m_b = mass of base = 250 g (density = 1 as it is a dilute solution), S_a = specific heat of acid = 1 (dilute solution), S_b = specific heat of the base = 1 (as it is also dilute), ω = water equivalent of the apparatus and t_a, t_b, t_m as determined by experimentations.

Calculate ΔH_{total} by substituting the value of Q in equation (2), ΔH_{total} is calculated and substituting the value of ΔH_{total} is equation (1), calculate the value of ΔH i.e. heat of ionization of acetic acid, ΔH_2 = 13600 cal/mole being known.

Experiment - 6

Determination of Solubility and Heat of Solution

The purpose of the experiment is to determine the heat of solution of succiric acid by measuring its solubility at three/four temperatures and applying the Van't Hoff equation to the data obtained. The Van't Hoff equation is expressed as :

$$\text{Log } S = -\Delta H / 2.303RT + C$$

Where, S is the solubility at temperature T, ΔH is the average heat of solution over the temperature range studied, R is the universal gas constant in calories per degree (K) per mole and a constant of integration. From this it can be seen that a plot of log S versus 1/T should be linear. Thus, ΔH and C can be determined from the slope and intercept of the plot on the Y-axis respectively.

The solubility may be expressed in grams or moles of solute per 100 g of the solvent.

Procedure:

A saturated solution (about 25-30 g in 100 mL) of succinic acid in water is prepared at about 50°C-55°C (A water batch is to be used). About 20 mL of the saturated solution is immediately poured into each of the three 100 mL. Erlenmeyer flask, sealed and placed in constant temperature baths, maintained at three pre-fixed temperatures (say 40°C, 50°C and 55°C). As the solutions cool, crystallization will take place. The solutions are shaken frequently and at the end of at least 15 minutes, 5 mL solution is withdrawn with a warm pipette (10 mL Mohr pipette) fitted with a Teflon plug to prevent the withdrawal of any solid succinic acid. The content of the pipettes i.e. the sample (5 mL) is discharged into a previously weighed weighing bottle, and weighed. The weighed sample is quantitatively transferred into a 250 mL conical flask, about 25 mL of water is added and titrated with a standard 0.5 N NaOH solution using phenolphthalein as the indicator.

If there is enough time left, each determination may be carried out in duplicate.

Calculations:

From the volume of sodium hydroxide consumed and its normality and known equivalent weight of succiric acid, the weight of the sample (succiric acid in each case) in grams per 100 g of water at the previously fixed temperature can be calculated for each temperature. Average value of duplicated determinations at the sample temperature is preferable. (Weight of the solute = V × N NaOH × milliequivalent).

i.e. ω_{solute} = wt of the sample solute in grams per the volume taken for titration

Then, weight of the solvent = $W_{soln.} - \omega_{solute}$

% of solubility, S, i.e. S% (w/w) = $100(\omega_{solute} / (W_{soln.} - \omega_{solute}))$

Log S vs.1/T is, now plotted on regular coordinate graph paper and the best-fitted straight line through the points is drawn. From the slope of the straight line the value of ΔH, the heat of solution is evaluated.

Also you may calculate the heat of N solution of salicylic acid from solubility measurements by calorimetric method.

Experiment - 7

Solubility and Qualitative Determination of Solubility Behavior

Many factors act to affect the extent and rate at which a solid drug dissolves into a solvent. This experiment will serve to illustrate some of these factors and produce in the student a more intuitive feeling of the process involved in the dissolution of drugs in pharmaceutical solvent systems.

The molecules in a solid drug are held together by certain intermolecular forces as induced dipole-induced dipole, dipole-dipole, and ion-ion interactions. Molecules of solvent are also associated by similar types of inter-molecular forces. We speak of solvents as being polar, semi-polar or non-polar depending on the magnitude of these molecular interactions.

In order for a solid to dissolve in a liquid or a liquid to mix with another liquid the intermolecular forces must be broken in each material and in general, new interactions must form between the two different materials before a solution can be formed. The extent to which dissolution or miscibility can take place depends upon the magnitude of force involved in these interactions. In general for dissolution to occur the forces of interaction between solute molecules and among solvent molecules must be less than forces of interaction between solute and solvent molecules. These solute-solvent interactions may be induced dipole-induced dipole, dipole-induced dipole, dipole-dipole, ion-dipole, etc.

We can briefly summarize these considerations by stating that qualitatively at least non-polar solutes are soluble in non-polar solvents and polar solutes soluble in polar solvents.

We also have available means other than alteration of solvent polarity for producing increased solubility of drug. The solubility of acidic or basic drugs may be altered by changing pH's (i.e. hydrogen ion concentration) of the solvent. Through the Law of Mass Action we, in effect, alter the polarity of our drug molecule to increase or decrease solubility by converting it between dissociated and un-dissociated forms.

Qualitative Determinations of Solubility Behavior

Reference: Merck Index; Mc Bluain, The characterization of Organic compounds, Chapter-3.

The experiment is designed to provide experience in determining and estimating the solubility characteristics of chemical compounds. A number of different chemicals will be provided. Their solubilities in water, ethyl alcohol, chloroform, 5% NaOH and 5% HCl are to be qualitatively determined. Generalizations concerning solubility relationships are to be made.

Procedure: 0.2 g (approximately) of a powdered solid is mixed with 10 mL of solvent in a test-tube, shaken vigorously and then examined for the presence of undissolved solid. In tabulating the results, the compounds provided are to be classified first into the following classes: weak acids, weak bases, phenolic compounds, strong electrolytes, and non-electrolytes. For each solvent investigated, solubility is to be denoted by a plus (+) sign, insolubility by a minus (–) sign after 2,5,10 and or 5 minutes.

Finally, by solubility tests, the chemical class of each of the unknown compounds supplied is to be determined.

The following compounds will be supplied: (at least five, each batch)

Benzoic acid	Quinine sulphate	Theophyllin
Phenol	Phenobarbital	Sulfadiazine
Quinine	Saccharin	Sucrose
Aspirin	Sodium Phenobarbital	Benzocaine
Acetanilide	Sodium chloride	Naphthalene

In your report write down the structure of each compound and indicate the group or groups responsible for solubility in the various solvent.

The student is expected to evaluate the results of these tests and formulate some generalities concerning the solubility characteristics of organic compounds.

Experiment - 8

Use of the Dielectric Constant – Solubility Relationship for Blending Pharmaceutical Solvent System

Introduction

The solubility of a solute in a solvent is usually related to the polarity of the solvent. More polar solutes require more polar solvents. Moreover, it can be shown that a polar solute has little tendency to dissolve in a non-polar solvent and vice versa.

The dielectric constant of a particular solvent, i.e. the effect that the solvent has on the ease of separation of two oppositely charged bodies placed within it, is related to its polarity and degree of association of its molecules. A series of solvents with gradually decreasing polarity will usually show the same progression in dielectric constant.

Table 8.1 Dielectric constants for some common Pharmaceutical solvents at 25°C

Solvent	λ*	Solvent	λ*
Water	78.5	Chloroform	4.8
Sorbital solution USP (70% w/w)	62.0	Castor oil	4.5
Syrup USP	56.0	Sesame oil	3.1
Glycerol	42.5	Olive oil	3.1
Propylene glycol	32.1		
Ethyl alcohol	24.3		
Acetone	20.7		
Iso-propyl alcohol	18.3		
Amyl alcohol	13.9		
Benzyl alcohol	13.0		
Polyethylene glycol-400	12.4		

[These values are from National Bureau of Standards Circular 514. "Table of Dielectric Constants of Pure Liquids". Alternatively, it can be determined experimentally with the help of Dielectrometer]

The value of the dielectric constant for a mixture of two or more liquids (*solvents) is often approximately equal to the sum of the products of the weight percent and dielectric constant of each individual component present. Mathematically, this can be expressed as:

$$D = \Sigma(\% (A)(\lambda_A) + (\% (B)(\lambda_B) + \ldots\ldots (-)$$

One can, thus, calculate the value of the approximate dielectric constant for a mixture by simple mathematical considerations. (The exact value can be ascertained, if required, by experimental method with the help of dielectric constant measuring instrument). The following example will serve to illustrate the method of calculations.

Example 1: What will be the dielectric constant for a 40% w/w* solution of ethanol in water? Using the values from the given table, we have:

$$24.3 \times 0.40 = 9.7$$
$$78.5 \times 0.60 = 47.1$$
$$56.8 \quad \text{i.e. } D = 56.8$$

*[%(w/w) are always used when calculating dielectric constants. Percent v/v is often more convenient: Weights and Volumes of pure liquids are inter-convertible when the specific gravity (and hence density) of liquids in question are known].

The curve shown clearly proves that the answer from our calculation is nearly identical to the experimentally determined values.

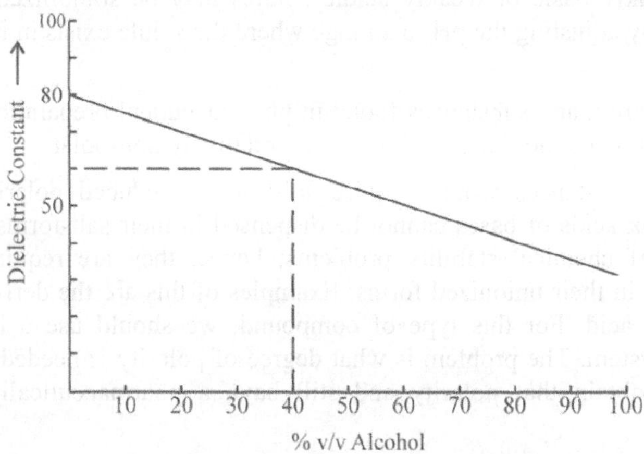

Fig. 8.1 Experimentally determined Dielectric Constant of Alcohol - Water Mixtures.

Experimentally Determined Dielectric Constants of Alcohol-water Mixtures

[This curve is reproduced from *Pharmaceutical Compounding and Dispensing*, R.A. Lyman. ed. Fig. 20, P-168]

It is also possible to calculate the relative proportions of two or more solvents needed to obtain a resultant mixture of desired solvents with a predetermined dielectric constant. This problem is most easily solved by using allegation, although an algebraic solution is also possible (See "Pharmaceutical Calculations", Bradley).

Example 2: In what proportions should one mix ethanol, glycerol and water to obtain a mixed solvent system having dielectric constant, D = 51.50?

Solvent	λ*	Parts by wt (Percent)	D
Water	78.5	40.00	31.40
Ethanol	24.3	30.00	7.29
Glycerol	42.5	30.00	12.75
			51.44

Now, how can we make practical use of this property of dielectric constants?

From consideration of solvent-solute interactions, one knows that polar solutes dissolve more easily in polar solvents while more non-polar solutes required non-polar solutes require non-polar solvents. We know also that some weakly basic or weakly acidic solutes may be solubilized in polar solvents by adjusting the pH to a range where the solute exists in its ionized form.

There are many substances found in pharmaceutical preparations which are neither acidic nor basic and which are relatively non-polar.

These substances would require solvents of reduced polarity. Also, some weak acids or bases cannot be dispensed in their salt-forms in water because of chemical stability problems; hence, they are required to be dispensed in their unionized forms. Examples of this are the derivatives of barbituric acid. For this type of compound, we should use a less polar solvent system. The problem is what degree of polarity is needed and how one can obtain that polarity and still have a pharmaceutically correct vehicle.

The problem of finding the correct degree or polarity (or non-polarity) is not extremely difficult to solve. Solutions are prepared containing varying concentrations of acetone and water or ethanol and water ranging from 0% to 100% water. The required amount of drug to produce the same concentration as is required for the finished product is dissolved in each solution. After reaching equilibrium the drug will have precipitated from solutions where the polarity is too high or too low for solubilization. Solutions of satisfactory polarity will show no precipitation. One can now, choose the solvent at the point where precipitation did not occur, as the solvent of choice.

The problem of obtaining a correct vehicle now arises. It may be necessary to mix certain solvents in such proportions that the polarity is approximately correct and at the same time, have a pharmaceutically elegant preparation.

As an example of the method of attack on this problem, let us take the case of a hypothetical drug (HA) which is a weak acid. It is unstable in aqueous solutions of high pH. Solubility product (S_o) is so low that precipitation is obtained at a low pH. However, we want to administer the drug in its dissolved form. The drug is highly soluble in alcohol. Now the prescription demands that we must have a solution containing the desired amount (say; 15 mg mL^{-1}) of final preparation.

Our first step is to determine what is the maximum polarity (dielectric constant); Which will allow dissolution of our drug at the prescribed dosage level? We would make solutions containing the drug in varying alcohol concentrations and observe them after a short period of time. The procedure for this type of study and the results are shown in the following table.

% w/w Ethanol ----	0	10	20	30	40	50	60	70	80	90
mL ethanol 90% w/w	-	1.3	2.6	3.8	5.0	6.1	7.2	8.1	9.0	9.8
mL water **	10	8.9	7.8	6.7	5.6	4.6	3.6	2.6	1.7	0.8
Precipitate mg drug	150	150	150	150	150	150	150	150	150	150

**Instead of adding these amounts of water it would be possible to add enough water (distilled/demineralized) to the specified amount of alcohol (IP) to make a total volume of 10 mL in each test tube.

The results indicate that at least a 50% w/w solution of ethanol in water is needed to dissolve the desired drug.

The 50% w/w ethanol-water solution would be the simplest preparation we could make. However, the vehicle would not be pharmaceutically elegant due to the high alcohol concentration. We can, however, determine the dielectric constant necessary for the dissolution of HA from the following information:

Method of calculation of Dielectric constant of a mixed solvent system

$$78.5 \times 0.50 = 39.3$$

$$24.3 \times 0.50 = 12.2$$

We, now, have the information that 50% w/w alcohol solution have a dielectric constant D = 51.5. Above this value of dielectric constant precipitation would theoretically occur, below it there is no precipitation. Thus, we should blend our solvents to approximate this value. We should note that in actual practice we might pick up a somewhat lower value of dielectric constant (Є) for our formulation. This would help to insure that we were not on the borderline of insolubility. That is, from the above solubility data we cannot tell whether precipitation would occur at 40% w/w or 41% w/w ethanol. We only know that it has occurred above 40% w/w ethanol.

Let us, now, see what we can do by using some glycerol in our formulation. This would allow us to decrease the alcohol content. We are to try to approximate a dielectric constant value of 51.5. The necessary calculations may be carried out by use of allegation, (Reference : Example 2 where this method has been exemplified) where we find that we need 30% w/w each of ethanol and glycerin and 40% (w/w) of water.

Considering the instability of our hypothetical drug in aqueous solution, the water content should be reduced in this vehicle which we are to formulate. How can this be done? The obvious way is to substitute some solvent with relatively high polarity for certain part of water, for example sorbitol solution USP/IP or syrup of official grade. These agents would also impart sweetness to our vehicle and make it smooth tasting.

Let us, now, reformulate our vehicle using sorbitol solution (official grade) in the formula in addition to the previously mentioned ingredients.

Table 8.2 Dielectric Constant value (λ) calculation of a mixed solvent system

Solvent	λ	Parts by wt (Percent)	% by wt.
Water	78.5	9.00	10.0
Glycerol	42.5	20.00	22.2
Ethanol	24.3	10.00	11.1
Sorbitol	62.0	(51.50)	56.7
		90.50 ≈ 90.00	100.00

And its dielectric constant is 51.0 (approximately)

Note: We could alligate this problem in another fashion too and still can produce a satisfactory vehicle.

This is one possible formula, there are others. According to our theory we can adjust these percentages to any value as long as we do not change the approximate dielectric constant of the resulting preparation.

It may often be necessary to reduce the concentration of one or more ingredients to a predetermined level and increase the others for reasons of stability, pharmaceutical elegance or availability of the drug to the physiologic system. Let us briefly consider how this is done.

Example: Let us say that in the formula of the vehicle for HA we want to decrease the glycerol content from 22.2% w/w to a minimum of 20% w/w and to substitute in its place some ethanol. The dielectric constant of glycerol is 42.5 of alcohol 24.3. Thus glycerol contains 42.5/24.3 times as many "dielectric units" per unit weight than alcohol. Thus we would need to substitute ethanol (42.5/24.3) × 2.2 = 3.8 parts by weight to make up for the decrease in glycerol content from 22.2% to 20%. Our formula would then be:

Table 8.3 Derivation of the Formula

Solvent	Parts by wt	% by wt
Water	9.00	≈ 9.50
Glycerol	20.00	≈ 21.0
Ethanol	13.80	14.50
Sorbitol	51.50	54.20
	94.30	99.20 ≈ 100.00

We should note that this does not give us exactly 20% w/w of glycerol content in the final formula.

A better way to approach this problem is to arbitrarily fix the percentage of a second component. For example water. Let us fix water content at 10.0% by weight**. Now, glycerol + water = 20.00 + 10.00 = 30.00% w/w in the total formula.

Ethanol + Sorbitol solution must therefore, make up the remaining 70.0% w/w of the total formula. The water and glycerin supply (0.10 × 78.5) + (0.20 × 42.5) ≈ 16.35 of the 51.50 dielectric constant units needed for the product. Thus, alcohol + sorbitol solution must supply the rest (51.50 – 16.35) = 35.15 units ≈ 35.00 units of dielectric constant.

Let the % w/w of ethanol be X and % w/w of sorbitol solution be Y. We have two unknown values. We know from algebra that in order to find out the values of X and Y we must set up and solve simultaneously two equations each relating X and Y.

**The following procedure requires that one of our variables must have a dielectric constant value greater than our final formula (here 51.50) and that the other must have a dielectric constant lower than the desired value (51.50). Thus we could not have fixed the alcohol concentration and allowed water and sorbitol solution to vary.

Since alcohol and sorbitor solution must supply 70.00% w/w of the total formula content we can write :

$$X/100 + Y/100 = 0.70 \qquad \text{.....(1)}$$

And since, they must supply 35 units of dielectric of dielectric constant, we can also write:

$$24.3X/100 + 62.0Y/100 = 35 \qquad .....(2)$$

And solving (1) and (2) simultaneously for X and Y we obtain : X = 22.28 ≈ 22.3% w/w and

$$Y = 47.7\% \text{ w/w}$$

The final formula will then be:

Table 8.4 The Final Formula

	% w/w
Water	9.50
Glycerol	21.00
Sorbitol, USP/IP	47.70
Alcohol, IP	22.30

One can visualize a large variety of formula manipulations of this type.

It should be noted here that while the discussion in this outline has been concerned with dissolving a non-polar solute in a mixed solvent system of maximum possible polarity the reverse situation may exist in some problems, i.e. the dissolution of a polar solute in a solvent of minimum polarity. The method of attack on this type of problem is identified.

Let us, now, make some comments regarding the validity of this method of using approximate dielectric constants to blend pharmaceutical solvents.

These calculated values of dielectric constant (λ) are only approximate. Complex formation and other interactions between the various components of the solvent will alter the dielectric constant value from the calculated one; likewise solvent-solute interactions of this type may increase or decrease solubility. The presence of electrolytes and other materials contained in the preparation may alter the solubility of the drug in the vehicle. These factors, among others, should be considered when formulating solvent systems using the dielectric constant method.

These deviations from the predicted values do not, however, negate the usefulness of this technique. Use of the dielectric constant property in blending a solvent system is a powerful tool. It gives us an intelligent and scientific method of attacking the problem of dissolving a drug in a pharmaceutically correct form. Since the method is quite simple and requires a minimum of equipment and materials, it may be applied to formulation of drug products or to problems in prescription compounding.

It is, therefore, a useful tool even for the retail pharmacists.

Reference: Moore, W.E., *J. Amer Pharm Assoc*, Sci. Ed, **47**, 855 (1958)

Procedure

The maximum polarity which will allow complete dissolution of the amount of the particular drug assigned is to be determined. The ethanol-water mixtures as explained in the experimental outline or any other desirable and suitable mixtures of non-polar-polar solvents may be utilized, calculating dielectric constant as also described earlier. The same may also be done for the polar-non-polar combination at which the solute just remains undisclosed.

1. The proportions of the following solvents required to give each the desired dielectric constant when combined is first calculated.
   (a) Ethanol-water-glycerin
   (b) Ethanol-water-sorbitol
   (c) Ethanol-water-sorbitol-glycerin (alcohol content must be less than 20%)
2. These solutions are prepared and to each of these mixtures is added the amount of drug previously utilized. It is then checked to see if the solubility or lack of solubility corresponds to the ethanol-water or previously observed results.
3. All calculations are to be shown in your report.

Experiment - 9

Measurement of pH and Buffer Solutions

Buffers are compounds or mixtures of compounds consisting of weak acids and their respective conjugate bases or vice-versa which, by their mere presence in solution, resist change in pH upon the addition of small quantities of acid or alkali. The resistance to a change in pH or H^+ ion concentration is known as buffer action.

The pH of a buffer solution and the change in pH upon the addition of an acid or a base may be calculated by the use of the buffer equation, known as the Henderson-Haselbalch equation. This equation is derived by considering, for example, the ionization of a weak acid such as acetic acid:

$$HAC + H_2O \rightleftharpoons H_3O^+ + AC^-$$

The equilibrium is described by the equilibrium constant :

$$K_a = [H_3O^+]\,[AC^-] / [HAC] = 1.8 \times 10^{-5}$$

Rearrangement of the equation yields: $[H_3O^+] = K_a \times [HAC]/[AC^-]$

Which logarithmically can be expressed as: $\text{Log}\,[H_3O^+] = \text{Log}K_a + \text{Log}\,[HAC]/[AC^-]$

Or $\quad pH = p^{K}{}_{a} + \log[AC^-] / [HAC]$

In general form, the buffer equation or the Henderson-Hasselbalch equation for a weak acid and its conjugate base (i.e. salt) is :

$$pH = pK_a + \log \frac{\text{Molar concentration of salt}}{\text{Molar concentration of the un - dissociated portion of acid}}$$

Thus, knowing the pK_a of the acid and the concentrations of salt and acid, the pH of such a solution can be calculated. Similarly, the composition of a buffer solution possessing a desired pH value can be calculated from the above relationship.

The magnitude of the resistance of a buffer to changes in pH by the addition of acid or alkali in small increment is referred to as the buffer capacity,

i.e. $\quad \beta = \Delta pH / \Delta V$

In which, β = buffer capacity, ΔpH = change in pH value by small increment, ΔV of acid or alkali.

Buffer capacity can, thus, be defined as the ratio of the increment of strong base (or acid) to the change in pH brought about by this addition. For example, the buffer capacity of a solution has a value of 1(one) when the addition of one gram-equivalent of a strong base or acid to a liter (IL) of the buffer solution results in a change of one pH unit. It can be reasoned that the buffer capacity of a buffer solution depends on the concentration of the buffer constituents and on the pH of the solution. The buffer is maximum at that pH where pH – pK_a= 0, i.e. the concentration of salt equals the concentration of the un-dissociated acid.

Note: Students are required to review the concepts of pH, pOH, pKw, as well as the use of the pH meter.

Procedure:

A. The directions for the use of the particular pH meter assigned to you in the laboratory must be followed carefully. Maximum care is to be adopted while handling the electrodes.

The pH meter is standardized first by using the standard pH-7-0-buffer provided. Then the pH of the following solutions is measured :

(a) standard pH-4.0 buffer
(b) 0.1 N acetic acid
(c) 0.1 N sodium salicylate
(d) 0.1 N ammonium chloride (NH_4Cl) solution
(e) 0.1 N ephedrine hydrochloride

The values obtained for b, c, d and e are, then, compared with the calculated values. Both the values (theoretical and practical data) are then tabulated in the report, explaining any differences, if observed).

B. Titration Curves

25.0 mL of 0.1 N HCl is measured out in a 100 mL beaker, 2 drops of phenolphthalein added and the pH of the solution is measured with the pH meter and recorded. The electrodes are lifted out of the solution, 2 mL of 0.1 N NaOH is added from a 50.0 mL burette and stirred with a small glass rod. [BE SURE NOT TO STIR WITH THE ELECTRODES IN THE SOLUTION]. Titration is continued with the addition of 2 mL increments of NaOH and each time pH reading is recorded until up to 22 mL is added. Then, the increments amount is reduced and reading noted each time until the exact end point is determined by the change of color from colorless to pink (in this case as phenolphthalein is the indicator).

[Why does this happen?]

This procedure is repeated using 1.0 mL increment of NaOH and no phenolphthalein, with:

(i) 25 mL of 0.1 N acetic acid
(ii) 25 mL of 0.1 N H_3PO_4

Titration curves are then drawn by plotting pH^- values on the Y-axis and mL of 0.1 N NaOH on the X-axis. The theoretical titration values for these systems are calculated at each addition (increment) point during titration and plotting these values on the same graph paper another titration curve is obtained.

[Discuss any differences you might observe]

C. Finally, using the stock solutions available a buffer of an assigned pH is prepared and its pH is measured and checked.

[**Note:** Once you have been assigned a task of preparing a buffer of a required pH, the amounts of buffer ingredients required to achieve the pH^- value are calculated and mixed. The pH of the prepared buffer solution is then measured to check the validity and the reliability of the procedure followed].

D. To verify the Ostwald's Dilution Law for a weak organic acid (say, acetic acid) using a pH-meter (Potentiometric method).

Apparatus and chemicals: A pH meter (A pH-meter which can indicate pH value in addition to the emf), acetic acid (or any assigned weak acid) solutions of 0.5 N, 0.25 N, 0.125 N and 0.0625 N and a standard buffer solution of known pH.

Ostwald's Dilution Law in mathematical form

$$K_a = \alpha^2 C/(1 - \alpha) = \alpha^2/(1 - \alpha)V$$

Procedure: The pH-meter will be ready for use only after 10-15 minutes' warming. After standardization with the buffer solution of known pH, the pH's of the prepared acid solutions are determined. From pH values $[H^+]$ concentrations are calculated using the equation, $pH = -\log_{10}[H^+]/c$ in case of each solution and finally $K_a = \alpha^2 C/(1 - \alpha)$. The mean of four reading yields, K_a, the dissociation constant of the acid.

E. To determine the pK_a value of a weak acid by titrating against strong base potentiometrically (using a pH-meter).

The required equation is: pH = pK_a + log[salt]/[acid] which is Henderson-Hasselbalch equation. (Halt-neutration process).

To discuss the exact end point plot of $\Delta pH/\Delta v$ vs V $\Delta pH/\Delta v$

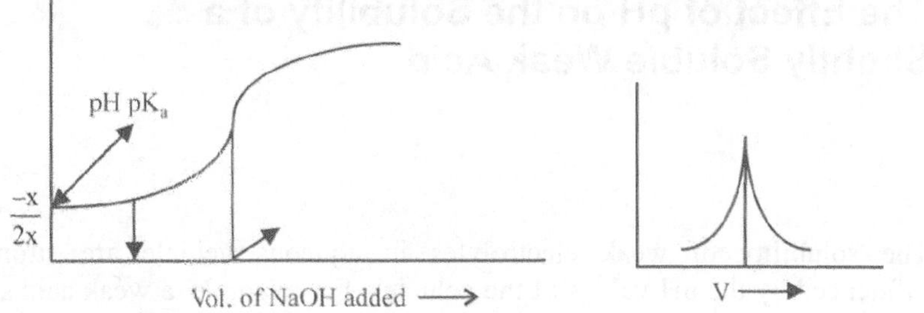

Fig. 9.1 Plot of Δ pH/ ΔV vs VΔ pH/ ΔV.

Experiment - 10

The Effect of pH on the Solubility of a Slightly Soluble Weak Acid

The solubility of weak electrolytes in aqueous vehicle are strongly influenced by the pH values of the vehicles. For example, a weak acid such as Phenobarbital has a relatively high solubility at pH values high in the alkaline region. When the pH of such a solution is lowered, the soluble ionic form is converted into the slightly soluble molecular form of Phenobarbital and the solution may exhibit precipitation. Similarly, weak bases such as various alkaloids are significantly more soluble at low pH values than at high-pH solution of alkaloidal salts, therefore, may exhibit precipitation when the pH of the medium is elevated.

The relationship existing between the solubility of a weak acid (or base) and the pH of the medium can be expressed as :

$$pH = pK_a + \log (S\text{-}S_0) / S_0$$

where, S = observed solubility at a certain pH

S_0 = Solubility in plain water

$pK_a = -\log K_a$ (K_a being the dissociation constant of a weak acid)

The experiment is designed to illustrate the effect of dissociation in the aqueous phase on the partition co-efficient of a weak acid. Salicylic acid is chosen as an example. The effect of pH on its distribution between water solution and benzene is to be investigated and also between buffer solutions and benzene which is desired in the required experiment.

Procedure:

Students will work in pairs:

A-1] An accurately prepared solution of sodium salicylate (40 mg mL^{-1}) is the first requirement. 5.00 mL of this solution is accurately pipetted out and delivered into a 100.00 mL volumetric flask and volume is adjusted with distilled water up to the mark. (Be very precise, since this solution will represent your standard solution). The standard solution prepared now represents a concentration of sodium salicylate equal to 2.00 mg mL^{-1}.

The following solutions are prepared

1. 5.00 mL of standard solution / 100 mL of solution
2. 10.00 mL of the standard solution / 100 mL of solution
3. 15.00 mL of the standard solution / 100 mL of solution
4. 20.00 mL of the standard solution / 100 mL of water
5. 25.00 mL of the standard solution / 100 mL of water

A-2] The quantitative determination of sodium salicylate is based on the determination of the purple color produced by the addition of ferric nitrate solution to the sample. The purple color produced will be quantitatively determined with a 'spectronic' spectrophotometer at 525 nm (millimicron) against a blank.

Six test solutions were prepared in six marked test tubes in the following manner:

Test Tube No.1 - 1 mL of the solution no. 1 + 2 mL of ferric nitrate solution + 5 mL of water

Test Tube No.2 - 1 mL of the solution no. 2 + 2 mL of ferric nitrate solution + 5 mL of water

Test Tube No.3 - 1 mL of the solution no. 3 + 2 mL of ferric nitrate solution + 5 mL of water

Test Tube No.4 - 1 mL of the solution no. 4 + 2 mL of ferric nitrate solution + 5 mL of water

Test Tube No.5 - 1 mL of the solution no. 5 + 2 mL of ferric nitrate solution + 5 mL of water

Test Tube No.6 - 6 mL of water + 2 mL of ferric nitrate solution

This solution i.e. of Test Tube No.6 will be used as your blank

Then, the absorbance of each solution is then determined and a plot of absorbance (A) vs mg. of sodium salicylate per mL is plotted. This "Beer plot" should yield a straight line with an intercept of zero.

A-3] The partition coefficient of salicylic acid between water and benzene is determined by placing exactly 25.00 mL of the solution in a 100/125 mL glass-stopper bottle, and exactly 25.00 mL of benzene is added to it. The stopper is put in its position and the bottle is shaken vigorously and intermittently for 10 minutes and then the bottle is placed on the working table and allowed to stand for sometime till the two immiscible phases separate out completely. 10.00 mL of the aqueous phase is next withdrawn. The salicylic acid concentration is determined after color development as previously described. The experiment is run in duplicate.

The concentration of salicylic acid in the benzene layer (phase) is then calculated by difference. Then, the partition coefficient as defined by the ***equation:***

$$K = \frac{(\text{Salicylic acid}) \text{ in benzene layer}}{(\text{Salicylic acid}) \text{ in aqueous phase}} \text{ is calculated.}$$

A-4] The procedure is repeated with 25.00 mL of each of the following buffer solutions:

pH = 3,4,5,6 and 7 in place of 25.00 mL of distilled water.

A-5] Partition coefficient versus pH values of the aqueous phase plot is next drawn.

Discuss the results

A-6] pH's vs log $S\text{-}S_o$ / S_o plot is finally drawn. Is this linear plot? If so, the pK_a of salicylic acid is determined from the "Y" – intercept.

Experiment - 11

Viscosity of Liquids

Resistance is offered when one part of a liquid is moved past another, the coefficient of viscosity being a measure of this internal friction or resistance to flow.

The viscosity of a liquid is usually measured by observing the rate of flow of the liquids through some form of capillary tube. For accurate viscosity determinations, a steady flow parallel to the axis of the tube must be maintained, and its rate must not exceed a certain value, which is dependent on the viscosity of the liquid and the radius of the tube.

The law that expresses the various flow of liquids through such tubes was first deduced by Poiseuille. The Poieusille's Law gives the relation between the co-efficient of viscosity, η, and the volume, V of a liquid flowing across the whole cross section of the tube in unit time, the pressure P, and the radius, r, length l, of the tube and t is the time. It is expressed as:

$$\eta = \frac{\pi r^4 P.t}{81V} \quad .....(1)$$

It is usually difficult to measure absolute viscosity of a liquid by this method but, relative viscosity (i.e.) the ratio of the viscosity of a liquid to that of some standard liquid such as water is easily measured. If one knows the absolute viscosity of the standard liquid, at the temperature of experiment, absolute viscosities of unknown liquids may be computed.

In a simple viscometer the pressure driving a liquid of viscosity η_1, through the capillary depends on the difference in the liquid levels, h, the density, p_1, and the acceleration due to gravity, g, and is given by the expression $h.p_1g$.

If exactly the same volume of a second liquid of viscosity, η_2 is introduced into the same tube (capillary), the driving pressure is $h.p_2.g$, where p_2 is the density of the second liquid.

From equation (1) the viscosity is proportional to the pressure and time of efflux for the same volume.

Hence: $\eta_1/\eta_2 = h.p_1.g.t_1 / h.p_2.g.t_2 = p_1t_1/p_2.t_2$ .....(2)

Therefore, η_2 (of exptl. Liquid) $= p_2t_2/p_1t_1\ x\eta_1$

Procedure:

The Ostwald Viscometers to be used are very fragile and should be treated with care, as directed. They must be thoroughly cleaned and dried before and after use.

The viscometer is clamped so that it is always exactly vertical. This is then placed into a thermostat. Exactly 5 mL (or 7 mL or 8 mL) of distilled (or dematerialized) water is added to the viscometer. A dust free rubber tube loosely plugged with cotton should be attached to the smaller tube, and the liquid is drawn up into the bulb above the upper mark. The water is then allowed to flow down through the capillary and the stop-watch is started when the meniscus passes the upper mark and stopped when the meniscus passes the lower mark. Four or five determinations for each liquid should be made and recorded. They should agree within + 2 seconds. These measurements should be repeated with:

(a) Acetone-water mixtures: 20, 40, 60, 80 mole per cent of acetone.

(b) Pure acetone

(c) Benzene

(d) An unknown liquid to be obtained from the instructor

Repeat the determinations with benzene or any other assigned liquid at 50°C and water at 50°C.

Note the relative effect of temperature on the viscosity of a polar and a non-polar liquid and compute the value of E_v (activation energy to initiate flow) in each case.

Calculations:

The relative viscosities are calculated using equation (2). Absolute values for water at the temperature of the experiment will be obtained from "Handbook of Physical Constants" by Langue (or any handbook on the subject). The absolute values for the various systems may then be calculated.

For the acetone-solutions plot relative viscosities on the Y-axis and mole per cent of acetone on the X-axis.

To determine the concentration of a given polymer (poly vinyl alcohol (cold water soluble) from the viscosity measurement using Oswald viscometer.

Procedure is the same as discussed already. The experimental liquids in this case are aqueous solutions of PVA of differing concentration starting from 40mg/100 mL to 50mg/100mL. Standard is D.M.Water and another solution of PVA of unknown concentration. Time of fall between two marks is determined using each solution and also determining their respective density values. The equations required are

$$\eta_2 = \frac{\rho_2 t_1}{\rho_2 t_1} \times \eta_1 \text{and } \eta_{sp} = (\eta_2 / \eta_0 - 1)$$

Where, η_0 = viscosity of the dispersion medium (water in this case)
η_1 = viscosity of water = 0.008 poise (given),
ρ_1 = density of water at Room temperature = 1 g/cm^3,
ρ_2 = density of PVA solution,
t_1 = time of flow of water,
t_2 = line of flow of any given solution and
η_{sp} = specific viscosity of the dispersion.

Graph: Plot η_{sp} vs concentration in mg/100 mL. For dilute solutions it is almost a straight line passing through the origin. The concentration of unknown PVA solution is then read from the graph by using the time of flow value of the unknown.

Experiment - 12

Surface and Interfacial Tension Measurement

The capillary-rise, drop-weight, drop-count and Du Noüy ring method of measuring surface tension may be used in this experiment.

In the capillary rise method, a capillary tube, with a fairly uniform bore, is immersed into a larger test tube containing the liquid to be measured. If the tube is clean, the liquid level in the capillary will rise above the level of the bulk liquid in the outer tube. The extent of this "capillary rise" depends on the surface tension of the liquid the rise increasing with increasing surface tension.

In the laboratory, the equation relating surface tension and capillary-rise is required to be derived and discussed. The equation is:

$$\gamma = h.r.d.g./2$$

where, γ = surface tension,
h = height i.e. rise in the inner tube,
g = the gravity constant, 980 cm/Sec^2,
r = radius of the capillary and
d = density.

The radius of the tube will be measured by using the known values of density of water and surface tension for water at the temperature of the experiment.

For water, $\gamma = 75.196 - 0.145t - 0.00024t^2$

where t = temperature of the experiment (in degree centigrade).

Substances to be measured

(a) Pure water,
(b) benzene
(c) ethyl alcohol, or
(d) any pure organic liquid

Procedure:

The capillary tube to be used is provided with engraved graduations. The liquid is poured into the outer tube to a level just above of the bottom of the capillary tube, when the capillary tube is stoppered into place. After allowing the system to come to a constant temperature, the liquid in the capillary is raised slightly by gently blowing into a tube treading to the outer tube, and then allowed to fall back to its original position. Then slight suction is applied, causing the liquid level in the capillary to fall. This is then allowed to return to the original position. In both cases the level will return to the original position if the capillary is cleaned and dried properly after every use.

The difference in the level of the liquid in the capillary and that in the outer container, in centimeters, is read on the scale, the bottom of the meniscus being read each time.

Four or five measurements should be made and the results averaged. The experimental liquids to be supplied may be either a benzene, toluene or xylene or an alcohol and in each case distilled water should be taken as the reference liquid.

Calculations:

1. Calculate the radius of the tube, in cm.
2. Calculate the surface tension of the assigned liquid (say benzene) and compare with values in the literature (Handbook of Physics and Chemistry).
3. Calculate the surface tension of your unknown sample.

Surface tension can also be measured by Drop-weight and Drop-count methods and also by using the tensiometer or 'ring' method. (Users are advised to read the operating instruction manual supplied with the instrument by the manufacturer so that they can operate the instrument most efficiently and effectively).

A. Drop-weight Method

Reference: Dutta – *Principles of Physical Pharmacy and Biophysical Chemistry* – Page 279-280

The size of a drop of liquid, issuing out from a capillary orifice is governed by the surface tension of the liquid and the radius of the capillary. Harkin and Brown found that the mass, m, of a drop of liquid falling from a capillary orifice (or tube) of radius, r, is governed by the relation:

$$m.g = 2\pi r.\ \gamma\ .\varphi$$

where φ = is a correction factor for the apparatus used. If the drops of different liquids are compared using the same apparatus, called **Stalagmometer,** the correction factor will be eliminated, or,

$$m_1 g/m_2 g = 22\pi r.\ \gamma_1\ .\varphi\ /\ 2\pi r.\ \gamma_2\ .\varphi$$

where, m_1 and m_2 are masses of a drop of two liquids and γ_1 and γ_2 their respective surface tensions.

Then, we get the required equation which is expressed as: $m_1/m_2 = \gamma_1/\gamma_2$

Now, knowing γ_1, m_1 and m_2, γ_2; the unknown surface tension of the second liquid can be computed.

Experimental: The stalagmometer tube is first thoroughly cleaned by chromic acid mixture ($K_2Cr_2O_7$ + Concentrated H_2SO_4), washed and dried. It is first filled by the liquid no.1 up to a fixed mark by sucking and then 20 to 30 drops are allowed to fall in a previously weighed weighing bottle. The weight of 1 drop is then determined. The experiment is repeated thrice to verify the reproducibility of the data and the mean value is taken.

The stalagmometer is again cleaned and dried and the whole experiment is repeated with liquid no.2. The weights, w_1 and w_2 thus found, divided by the number of drops of each liquid give the weight of each drop, m_1 and m_2, respectively.

If the surface tension of one liquid is known, the surface tension of the other liquid can be calculated.

Room temperature is to be noted, Room temperature = __°C

Surface tension of distilled water at room temperature = 72 dynes/cm (to be corrected if the temp. is either higher or lower than 25°C)

B. Drop-Count Method for Surface and Interfacial Tension Measurement

Reference: Dutta – Principles of Physical Pharmacy & Biophysical Chemistry, Page 280-281

In this method, known (i.e. fixed) volumes of liquids are allowed to fall down from the same stalagmometer. The number of drops of each liquid falling from equal volume of each of them is then counted. Knowing the density and surface tension of one liquid and also the density of the second, the surface tension of the second liquid, the surface tension of the second liquid also the interfacial tension between the two liquids can be calculated.

We know, $m_1 = V_1d_1$ and $m_2 = V_2d_2$ where V_1 is the volume of a drop of liquid 1, d_1 the corresponding density and m_1 is the mass of the drop, V_2, d_2 and m_2 are the corresponding values for the second liquid.

Now, $m_1/m_2 = \gamma_1/\gamma_2 = V_1d_1/V_2d_2 = \dfrac{(V/\eta_1).d_1}{(V/\eta_2).d_2} = \eta_2.d_1/\eta_1.d_2$

For surface tension determination of the experimental liquid distilled water being used as the reference standard liquid.

The modified equation: $\gamma_1/\gamma_2 = \eta_2.d_1 \,/\, \eta_1.d_2 = \eta_2.d_1 \,/\, \eta_1(d_1 - d_2)$ is applied for the determination of the interfacial tension of the second liquid in the first one.

In practice, the liquids are allowed to drop from the upper marks to the lower marks (pre-fixed) and the number of drops counted in each case.

In the drop-count method the usual practice is to measure the volume, in preference to the weight of the drop. The apparatus generally is a stalagmometer or a pipette with the tip bent.

The number of drops produced by a definite volume of liquid in air in the first case and then in the lighter liquid is counted. Each time the number of drops falling out of the capillary tip (grounded base) emptying the prefixed volume is counted. The interfacial tension is computed by the use of the equation:

$$\gamma_{1,2} = \gamma_1 .\ \eta_1(d_1 - d_2)/\ \eta_2.d_1$$

Where,

$\gamma_{1,2}$ = the interfacial tension existing at the interface of the two immiscible liquids

γ_1 = surface tension of the standard (here water) at the temperature of the experiment

η_1 = number of drops of the heavier liquid (generally distilled water) in air and η_2 into the lighter liquid taken in a beaker emptying the same volume as in the previous case.

d_1 = density of the heavier liquid at the temperature of the experiment

and d_2 = density of the second liquid at the same temperature

The detergent action of soap and certain other cleaning agents is due to the lowering of the interfacial tension between water and the oil or greasy material to be removed.

The interfacial tension also plays a very important role in certain phenomena associated with the living cells.

C. Du Noüy ring method:

Surface and Interfacial tensions can also be measured using the tensiometer or "ring" method. The operating instructions are required to be carefully read so that the instrument is handled most effectively.

Preparing the instrument for use: The tensiometer is used for measuring small forces. The instrument being a very delicate one should be handled carefully and thoughtfully. It is to be kept in clean and operating condition after every operation, when not in use it is to be kept in the case.

The platinum ring must be handled carefully. To obtain accurate results the ring must be clean and in good condition. The ring must be kept in one place and the round shape (circle of uniform radius) must be preserved.

With reasonable care the instrument should last for many years. It is expected that replacement rings will be needed – the frequency of replacement depending upon the mode of use and care while handling the ring.

Both instruments (the tensiometer and the ring) are calibrated so that the dial reading is the apparent surface tension expressed in dynes per centimeter. If a known weight, M, is placed on the ring and balanced by the torsion in the wire, then the dial reading, p, is given by the equation.

$$P = mg/2L \qquad .....(1)$$

Where, m = weight expressed in grams
g = value of gravity in cm/sec^2
L = mean circumference of the ring in cm
P = dial reading = apparent surface tension in dynes/cm

The instrument is removed from the wooden case and placed on a level and stable bench free from vibration. A spirit level is placed on the sample table and is leveled until the level indicates the sample table is horizontal.

The instrument is shipped with the wire taut and in approximate adjustment as regards calibration. Further, adjustment now consists of an exact calibration so that the dial reading will indicate directly in dynes per centimeter. This exact calibration is accomplished by adjusting the length of the torsion arm.

The torsion arm is clamped with the adjustable stops. The dry ring (platinum ring) is placed in its position on the hook and a small strip of paper is cut into a suitable size and fitted on the ring as a platform. The torsion arm is released. The knurled nob is turned until the index and its mirror image are exactly in line with the reference line on the mirror. The dial clamp is loosened and the dial rotated until the vernier indicates approximately zero. The dial clamp is tightened and the dial rotated by means of the fine adjustment until the reading on the vernier is exactly zero.

On the paper is placed some accurately known weight from 500 mg to 800 mg and the knurled knob is turned until the index is again opposite and the reference line on the mirror. The dial reading is recorded up to 0.01 divisions.

Assuming that a weight of 600 mg is used, and then from the above equation (eqn.1) is determined what the dial reading and hence the surface tension should be. As an example:

$$m = 600 \text{ mg} = 0.600 \text{ g}$$

L = 6.00 cm (using the value given on the box by the manufacture)

$G = 980.3 \text{ cm/Sec}^2$

Then $$P = mg/2L = \frac{0.600 \times 980.300}{2 \times 6.000} = 49.01 \text{ dynes/cm}$$

If the recorded dial reading is greater than this calculated value, re-adjustment is made by shortening the torsion arm. If the dial reading is less the torsion arm is to be lengthened and again adjustment is done. The calibration procedure is repeated readjusting the zero position with paper-piece in place after each change until the dial reading agrees with the calculated value. Each unit on the dial then represents a surface tension of exactly one dyne per centimeter.

When the calibration is completed, the paper is removed from the ring and readjustment to zero position is done. To readjust the zero position the knurled knob is turned until the index and its mirror image are exactly in line with the reference line on the mirror, the dial clamp is loosened and the dial rotated until the vernier is approximately on zero. The clamp is tightened and the dial rotated with the fine adjustment screw until the vernier is exactly on zero position.

Procedure and determination of Apparent Surface Tension and Interfacial Tension:

In making surface and interfacial tension measurements one of the most important points is the cleanliness of the ring and the vessels/ The cleaning procedure recommended when testing oils (insulating or otherwise) is as follows. "Glassware is cleaned by removing any residual oil with benzene followed by several washes with methyl ethyl ketone and water and immersion in a hot cleaning solution of chromic acid followed by through washings with tap water and then with distilled water. The platinum ring is cleaned by rinsing it in benzene followed by rinsing in methyl ethyl ketone. It is then heated in the oxidizing portion of a gas flame". Only that portion of the ring which will be immersed in the liquid under test is to be heated. To obtain repeat values the ring must be cleaned between each determination.

For other material other suitable cleaning methods may be necessary and perhaps a less elaborate cleaning procedure may suffice. For accurate work all glass-ware and the ring must be chemically clean.

The calibration of any tensiometer should be checked periodically, especially each time the instrument is used after a period of idleness. In the following outline of operational procedures it is assumed that the instrument has been calibrated and is in adjustment.

(a) ***Surface tension measurement:*** To make a measurement of surface tension the cleaned and dried ring is attached to the lever arm. The liquid to be measured is placed in a clean and dry vessel such as a petri dish, watch glass (flat) or beaker at least 4-5 cm in diameter and the container placed on the sample table. With screw in its upper most position the entire sample table assembly is raised until the ring is immersed probably 5 mm in the liquid. Then, the entire assembly is lowered until the ring is just below the surface of the liquid and approximately centered with respect to the container. The liquid is further lowered by means of screw until the ring is in the surface of the liquid and the index is approximately on zero.

The torsion of the wire is increased by rotating the knob and at the same time lowering the sample table by means of screw so as to keep the index on zero. The index is to be kept on zero even though the surface of the liquid is distended. This double movement is continued until the film breaks.

The scale reading at the breaking point of the film is the apparent tension, p.

(b) ***Interfacial tension measurement:*** Interfacial measurements that can be made with an upward pull may be made with this instrument. The accepted practice is to mark the ring from water into the other liquid.

Ordinary adjustments are the same as for surface tension measurements. In raising or lowering the liquid rough adjustments are made by means of the screw.

When the measurement is to be made on the interface between water and a liquid lighter in density than water the ring pull is upward and the procedure is as follows:

With water in the clean dish, the platform is raised until the ring immersed from 5 to 7 mm in the water. A quantity of the liquid, immiscible with water, is then carefully poured on the surface of the water. This should be to a depth of 5 to 10 mm depending upon the liquid but deep enough to prevent the ring from entering the upper surface before the film breaks. The position of the dish is adjusted until the ring is in the interface and the lever arm in the neutral position. The torsion of the wire is increased and the dish lowered, keeping the index of the lever arm at zero. The reading when the film at the interface breaks is the apparent interfacial tension, $\gamma_{1,2}$.

The apparent surface tension and interfacial tension determined by the instrument, tensiometer, is to be corrected by multiplying with a correction factor provided by the manufacturer in the operating manual.

To Be Given In Class

It is necessary to know the ratio of the radius of the ring to the radius of the wire. The data, R/r, is furnished by the maker of the ring. It is also necessary to know the values of p, D and d. In this case p is the apparent surface (or interfacial) tension or reading on the tensiometer. When making a surface tension measurement, D is the density of the liquid and d is the density of the saturated air. When making an interfacial measurement, D, is the density of the lower liquid and d is the density of the upper liquid. In case of surface tension, d, the density of the saturated air is so small that in comparison to the density of most liquids that it may be ignored. Therefore, to determine the correction factor, f, the formula p/(D-d) may be used.

Systems to be measured

(a) Surface tension of water, benzene, mineral oil and oleic acid (make corrections), toluenes, xylene etc.

(b) Interfacial tension of water against oleic acid and mineral oil, benzene. Compare these values and calculate the work of cohesion and adhesion. Calculate the work of adhesion and hence, spreading co-efficient for mineral oil and oleic acid on water, and also of benzene on water.

(c) Compare the surface tension values of benzene obtained by the capillary, drop-weight and ring methods.

D. Calculate of the PARACHOR VALUE of the experimental liquid:

The formula for calculation of Parachor [P] of the liquid is : [P] = Parachor = M/D. $\gamma^{1/4}$ = c (a constant) × M and also [P] = $\gamma^{1/4}.V_M$,

Where, $M/D = V_M$ (molar volume of the liquid), M = Molecular mass of the liquid and d is its density.

Note: A molar volume is an additive property; Parachor is also an additive property in more accurate form.

Report the $[PCH_2]$ contribution towards the parachor value using the relations

$$[PCH_2] = [P]_{xylene} - [P]_{toluene};$$

Also, $[PCH_2] = [P]_{toluene} - [P]_{benzene}$

$$[PCH_2] = [P]_{ethanol} - [P]_{methanol} = [P]_{n\text{-}propanol} - [P]_{ethanol}$$

$$[P]_{isomeric\ branching} = [P]_{iso\text{-}propanol}$$

$$[P]C_6H_{14} - 6[P]_{CH2} = 2[P]_H,$$

therefore, $[P]_H$ can be calculated and finally,

$$[P]_C = [P]CH_2 - 2[P]_H$$

n-hexane, In this way, parachor contributions of each atom of a molecule in a particular configuration can be evaluated.

Experiment -13

Determination of the Critical Micelle Concentration (CMC) of a given Surfactant by Surface Tension Method

Apparatus:

Chemicals: Stalagmometer, any given surfactant of known molecular weight.

Procedure:

The procedure for determining surface tension of the surface-active agent will be the same as described in the previous experiment only difference being use of surfactant solutions of various concentrations.

Note: The stalagmometer need not to be dried every time. Only "rinsing" it with the desired solution of the surfactant solution each time is required.

Observations

Room temperature: = ... °C

γ_w = Surface tension of water at room temp,

d_s = density of the solution used each time

and d_w = density of water at room temperature or value of 1.0 g / mL may be taken as approximation.

Table 13.1 Change of surface tension w.r.t. change in concentration of solution

Liquid No.	C (mg%w/w)	No. of drops (n)				γ surface tension	d_n	d_c	d_n/d_c
		(i)	(ii)	(iii)	Mean				
1. (water)	0								
2.	5.00								
3.	10.00								
4.	20.00								
5.	30.00								
6.	50.00								
7.	60.00								
8.	80.00								
9.	100.00								

Calculations:

C = Concentration of surfactant solution in mg/100 mL in distilled water

Surface tension of the liquid, $\gamma_S = d_s/d_w \times n_w/n_s$

Where, γ_S = surface tension of the respective surfactant solution

d_s = density of the respective experimental solutions

d_w = density of distilled water at room temperature

n_w = number of drops of water

n_s = number of drops of experimental solutions

γ_w = surface tension of water at room temperature

d_n = difference in the no. of drops of two consecutive solutions

d_c = difference in the conc. of two consecutive solutions

and $d\,\gamma_S/d_c$ is the change in surface tensions of the surfactant solutions with change in concentration.

Graphs:

1. Surface tension vs. concentration plot is drawn. Two "extreme" tangents are drawn to the graph obtained. The point of intersection of the two tangents gives the critical micellar concentration (cmc).
2. In most cases it is difficult to draw tangents and hence the first derivative plot dn/dc *vs* concentration may be used to determine the cmc value (Figures are shown below):

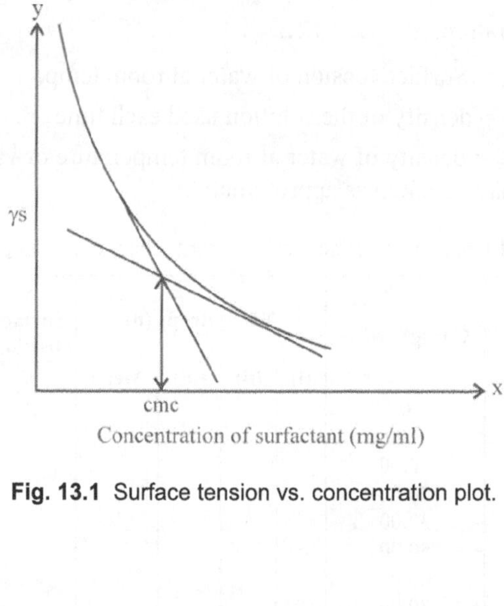

Fig. 13.1 Surface tension vs. concentration plot.

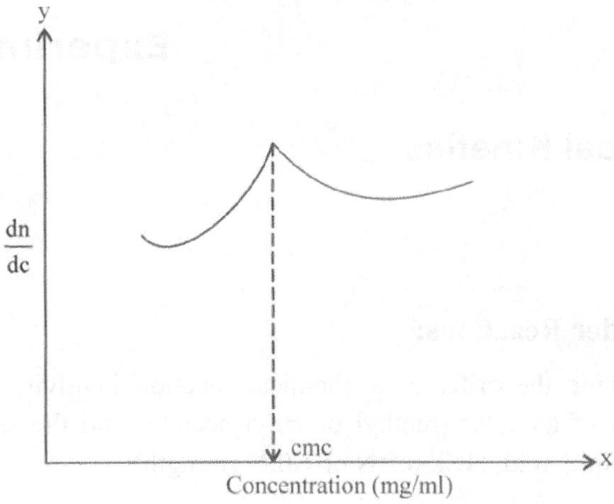

Fig. 13.2 $\frac{dn}{dc}$ vs. concentration plot.

Note: C_{mg}/100 mL = [(C_{mg}/M) × 10] mole/L where M = Molecular weight in grams.

Result: The critical micelle conc. of the surfactant

Solution = ... mg/100 mL

Or = ... mole/L

Precautions while using Stalagmometer:

1. Stalagmometer must be made clean and dried before every use.
2. It should be clamped in vertical position
3. Drop falling rates should be made slow so that the drop gets detached under its own weight.
4. Drop correction must be made by observing the meniscus carefully
5. While using the surfactant solutions of differing concentrations the stalagmometer may rinsed with the respective experimental solutions before taking reading and foaming should be avoided while handling surfactant solutions.

Experiment – 14

Chemical Kinetics

First Order Reactions:

To determine the order of a chemical reaction involving acid-catalyzed hydrolysis of an ester (methyl or ethyl acetate) and the specific reaction rate-constant (Acid, HCl, 0.5 N or 1.0 N strength).

When the rate of a reaction is dependent on the concentration of one species of the reacting molecules, we are dealing with first-order kinetics. Generally, for hydrolysis of esters, such an order will be followed since the concentration of water essentially remains constant throughout the reaction, while the ester concentration changes. Such reactions although actually bimolecular (ester + water), are known as pseudo-first-order reactions. In the presence of a constant hydrogen ion concentration, the rate will be accelerated, but the reaction will remain pseudo-first-order as H^+ will act as the catalyst.

The system to be studied is the acid-catalyzed hydrolysis of either methyl acetate or ethyl acetate or any other ester which will be available in the laboratory. The reaction is :

$$\text{Ester} + H_2O + [H^+] \xrightleftharpoons{\text{HCl}} \text{corresponding alcohol} + \text{parent acid} + [H^+]$$

$$\underset{\text{methyl acetate}}{CH_3COO\text{-}CH_3} + H_2O + [H^+] \xrightleftharpoons{\text{HCl}} \underset{\text{acetic acid}}{CH_3COOH} + \underset{\text{methanol}}{CH_3OH} + [H^+]$$

or

$$\underset{\text{ethyl acetate}}{CH_3COO\text{-}C_2H_5} + H_2O + [H^+] \xrightleftharpoons{\text{HCl}} \underset{\text{acetic acid}}{CH_3COOH} + \underset{\text{ethanol}}{C_2H_5OH} + [H^+]$$

The appearance of acetic acid will be followed as the reaction proceeds by removing samples at different time intervals and titrating with standard base.

Procedure:

100 mL of 1 N, HCl is placed into a 150 mL Erlenmeryer flask clamped in a constant temperature water-bath. Some methyl or ethyl acetate is placed in a separate container placed in the same temperature bath.

After allowing 10-15 minutes for temperature equilibrium exactly 5.0 mL of the ester is pipette out and put into this flask containing the acid. Time (t = 0) is noted. It is then shaken for thorough mixing; a sample of exactly 5.0 mL is then withdrawn immediately and run into 50 mL of ice-cold water (to arrest the reaction). The time at which the pipette has been half-emptied into the water of the titration flask is recorded along with the titration - using 0.2 N NaOH solution. Three more samples are removed and titrated at 10-minutes intervals, then at 20,30,40 and 60 minutes intervals for the rest of the laboratory period shaking is needed before each withdrawal. Twenty four hours later a final sample (5.0 mL) is removed and titrated with the same (0.2 N NaOH) solution. This represents the completed reaction. Alternatively, the reaction mixture may be refluxed for 1 hr. and then cooled to room temperature before the final titration.

You plan your work so that you can also run samples at 35°C, 45°C and 50°C (3-4 laboratory days may be required to complete the plan-programme).

Calculation:

The difference between the titration values at any time, t, and at the end of 24 hours (or after boiling and cooling of the reaction mixture), when the reaction is assumed to be completed, is a measure of the concentration of the ester that remains unhydrolyzed at time, t, viz. ($T_t - T_0 = X$) and ($T_\infty - T_0$) = a.

Each molecule of ester produces one molecule of acid (in this case acetic acid) and the increase in acidity is, therefore, due to the amount of the ester (acetate) that has reacted ($[H^+]$ concentration of HCl solution remains constant).

The concentration of acetate at various times is plotted against time, time as the independent variable (X-axis) and concentration as the dependent variable (Y-axis).

A second plot of log concentration vs. time is also drawn and if the system is first-order a straight line should be obtained. From this straight-line curve, the specific reaction rate-constant is computed. From the rate constant the half life ($t_{½}$) for the reaction is calculated.

Having calculated the rate-constant, K, at three more pre-determined temperatures (using a thermostatic bath) and applying the Arrhenius equation ($k = A.e^{-Ea/RT}$) by plotting log k versus 1/r, the corresponding frequency factor, A, and the energy of activation, E_a, are determined.

Data: Reaction temperature (water bath thermostatic) = ...°C

Titre at zero time, t = 0 is T_0, at time, t = T_t = ... and titrate at infinity, $t_\infty = T_\infty$ = ... mL of 0.2 N NaOH.

Initial concentration of the ester, a = $T_\infty - T_o$ = ... mL of 0.2 N and unhydrolyzed ester concentration at time, $t_\infty(T_\infty - T_t)$ = ... mL of standard 0.2 N NaOH.

Observation:

Time, t (in min)	Titre, T_t	Amount reacted, $x_\infty(T_t - T_o)$	Amount remaining un-reacted (a – x) $\infty(T_\infty - T_t)$	Log_{10} (a-x)	Specific rate constant, k in min^{-1}
Initial T_o time					(nil)
10					
20					
30					
50					
80					
120					
180					
Infinity reading T_∞					(nil)
					Mean value of k =........ min^{-1}

Equation to be used :

1. $t = 2.303/k \times \log_{10} a/(a - x)$

   Or $\log_{10}(a - x) = - kt/2.303 + \log_{10} a$

2. Plotting $\log_{10}(a\text{-}x)$ vs t, a straight is obtained (for the first order reaction) yielding a negative slope, – k/2.303 = (-) slope, therefore, k = (2.303) (slope value) min^{-1}
3. By plotting x *vs* t, a curve will be obtained
4. Arrhenius equation, $k = A.c^{-Ea/RT}$ or log k = log A –(Ea/2.303.RT)

therefore, plot of log k against 1/T also will result in a straight line with a slope n (-ve) = (– Ea/2.303R) from which Ea is computed.

To determine the relative strengths of two acids HCl and H_2SO_4 kinetically

Procedure, chemicals, apparatus set up. Calculation, graphs etc. are all same as in the previous experiment (experiment No.14.1); only difference is that in place of HCl (1.0 N), H_2SO_4 (1.0 N) is used as the catalytic agent.

Let the specific reaction rate constant in case of H_2SO_4 be K_{H2SO4} and that of HCl be k_{HCl}.

Result: the relative strength of the two acids = K_{H2SO4} / K_{HCl}

To determine the half-life period ($t_1/2$) for the above-discussed first-order reaction

For a first order reaction $t_{½}$ is independent of concentration and is expressed as $t_{½} = 0.693/k$. By determining $t_{½}$ of the reaction, k, specific rate constant can be determined.

Calculation of Energy of Activation, Ea in Kcal mole^{-1}. Energy of activation is computed from the Arrheniees equation : $k = A.e^{-Ea/RT}$

At temperature T_1 K, $k = A.e^{-Ea/RT}{}_1$ and at temp. T_2 K; $k = A.e^{-Ea/RT}{}_2$, where R = gas constant,

= 1.987 cal deg.$^{-1}$ mole^{-1}, A = frequency factor, and T is the temperature (in Kelvin scale) at which reaction is performed.

Therefore, $l_n(k_2/k_1) = E_a/R(1/T_1 - 1/T_2)$

Or $\log(k_2/k_1 = E_a/2.303R \times (T_2\text{-}T_1)/T_1T_2$

Or $Eq = 2.303\ R.T_1T_2 \log(k_2/k_1)/(T_2 - T_1)$

Experiment – 15

Chemical Kinetics Involving Second-order Reactions

When the velocity of a reaction is dependent on the concentrations of two reacting species the rate of the reaction may be expressed as follows :

$$rate = dx/dt = k_2(a-x)(b-x) \quad .....(1)$$

Where, k_2 is the reaction rate constant of second order reaction : A+B C+D, and a and b are the initial concentrations of the reacting substances. Let, x be the amount of each which has been consumed in time, t.

Now, two cases may arise (i) when a and b are originally equal, the equation becomes :

$$dx/dt = k_2\,(a-x)^2 \quad .....(2)$$

This upon integration yields:

$$k_2 = 1/a.t\,.\,x/(a-x) \quad .....(3)$$

And (ii) when $a \neq b$; the form of the equation (1) becomes : $dx/dt = k_2(a-x)(b-x)$

Generally, in the laboratory procedure the reacting species are taken in equal quantities and hence the integrated form of the equation number (3) is applicable and is used to compute k_2, the second-order specific reaction rate constant. Processes fitting such a relationship are known as second-order reactions.

The reaction to be studied is the saponification of an ester such as ethyl acetate :

$$CH_3COOC_2H_5 + NaOH \rightleftharpoons CH_3COONa + C_2H_5OH$$

In this experiment, the loss of OH^- with time will be followed either by titration method using standardized HCl solution or conductometrically. We are taking advantage of the very high conductance of OH^- as compared to the acetate ion which is formed. The following equation equivalent to eq.3 is applicable in the case.

$$k_2 = 1/t\,(A - E).[(A - T)/(T - E)] \quad .....(4)$$

where, A – represents the initial conductance,

E, the final conductance (24 hours later) and T, is the conductance at time t.

Procedure:

First, a 0.1 N standard NaOH solution in distilled water is prepared (100 mL) from this 10 mL is taken out and it is diluted to 100 mL to get a 0.01 N NaOH solution. It is then placed in the conductance cell and its conductance is measured. This value is A. The conductance cell is then rinsed with distilled water to remove all traces of NaOH.

Then from the standardized NaOH solution (stock solution of 0.1 N), 100 mL of 0.02 N solution of NaOH is prepared. This container containing 0.02 N NaOH and another container containing 0.02 N ethyl acetate solution are placed into the thermostat. Temperature is noted or adjusted as needed.

When temperature equilibrium is established, at an observed time, 50 mL of 0.02 M(=N) NaOH is mixed with exactly 50 mL of 0.02 M(=N) ester and the mixed solution is placed into the conductivity cell after quickly rinsing the cell with a small portion of this first. The time of mixing marks the start of the reaction which is noted.

Conductance is measured every minute for the first 10 minutes, every 5 minutes for the next 20 minutes, 10 minutes intervals up to an hour and then every 15 months. The final reading will be made next day.

Calculations:

1. Observed conductance is plotted against time, t
2. 10 points are selected (or picked up) ranging from the beginning to the end of the period and T vs (A – T)/t is plotted. If the plot is linear, the relationship is second order, since it follows the following equation which is equation 4 rearranged.

$$t = 1/k_2(A - E)[\,(A - T)/(T - E)]$$

The slope will equal $1/k_2.a$ and the intercept on the Y = axis is E (1) compare this value of E with that obtained after 24 hours, (2) calculate k_2 from the slope.

Experiment - 16

Conductivity of Solutions

Electrons are negatively charged particles and they carry a negative charge and the flow of electrons through metallic conductors is called electric current. The passage of electric current through the solution is primarily due to the movement of ions between the electrodes. The Ohm's Law V = IR is applicable to both the metallic conduction as well as the solution conduction.

Where,

V = potential difference (in volts) between the two ends of the conductor

I = current in ampere

R = resistance (Ohm)

The resistance, R, of the metal or the solution depends on the length, l, of the metal conductor or the solution column length between the two electrodes and also on the cross-sectional area, A, of the conductor or of the solution column. Hence,

R ∞ l/A or R = p.l/A, therefore, p = R.A./l and C=1/R = 1/P.A/l = k.A/l = Ohm.cm^2/cm = Ohm cm, where C (current) i.e. conductance of the solution (or metal) P = specific resistance of the metal or the solution and k (Kappa) = specific conductance of the metal or the solution. In C.G.S. Units : P = Ohm. cm; k(kappa) = 1/p = $Ohm^{-1}cm^{-1}$ = mho.cm^{-1}

Specific Resistance of a material in solution is defined as the resistance offered by 1 cm^3 of that material when placed between two parallel electrodes 1 cm apart.

Specific conductance of a material is defined as the conductance of 1 cm^3 of the material when placed between two parallel electrodes 1 cm apart.

Equivalent Conductance "λ" (lamda) of a solution is defined as the conductance of a volume of solution containing 1g equivalent weight of the solute when the whole of the solution is placed between two parallel electrodes 1 cm apart.

λ = k.V, where, k = specific conductivity (or conductance)

and V = volume in cm^3 (or mL) containing 1g equivalent weight of the solute.

Units of $\lambda = Ohm^{-1}\ cm^2$

If C is the concentration of a solution in gram equivalents per liter, the concentration per cm^3 is C/1000 and the volume containing 1 equivalent of the solute is, therefore, $1000/C.cm^3$. Since, k, is the specific conductance, i.e. the conductance of 1 cm^3 of the solution, the conductance of $1000/C.cm^3$ solution, and hence,

$$\lambda \text{ (equivalent conductance)} = 1000\ k/C$$

The above equation is the defining expression of the equivalent conductance. It must be noted that C in this equation is in equivalents of solute per liter of solution.

When molar concentration is considered the above equation also gives a measure of molar conductance, λ_M

Degree of Dissociation: (α)

Degree of dissociation, α, is defined as the fraction of an electrolyte that dissociates in aqueous solution. For strong electrolyte, dissociation is almost complete at any moderate concentration. But for weak electrolytes, the degree of dissociation, (α) is very low. But, on dilution, (α) goes on increasing and at very high dilutions (i.e. at infinite dilution) the degree of ionization is almost complete i.e. $\alpha \sim 1$. The equivalent conductance, λ. of the solution of a weak electrolyte also goes on increasing with dilution and is practically constant at a very high dilution condition, and is called equivalent conductance at infinite dilution, λ_∞.

Conductivity cell: A conductivity cell consists of two parallel inert electrodes (usually platinum electrodes coated with platinum black) separated by a fixed distance, l, inside a glass cylinder. The electrodes, each having the same area, A, may be circular or rectangular.

Cell constant: The ratio of l/A is called the cell constant, Unit of cell constant is cm^{-1}

Experiment - 16A

To Determine the Cell Constant of a Given Conductivity Cell

Apparatus:

Conductivity Meter, Conduct metric Cell.

Chemicals: 0.02 N KCl solution of known specific conductance = 0.003 mho cm^{-1} = 3.00 milli mho/cm at 25°C.

Procedure:

The conductivity cell is washed thoroughly with distilled water and the cell is then made dry with the help of filter paper strips.

The cell electrodes are then dipped into the prepared 0.02 N KCl solution which must be sufficient enough to cover the whole of the electrodes.

The temperature Knob is adjusted to read the temperature of the solution and the conductance of the solution is used by selecting the appropriate (Knob) range.

Calculation:

If the observed conductance is k_o for the 0.02 N KCl solution in milli mhos.cm^{-1} then true specific conductance = Observed conductance x cell constant.

Therefore, Cell constant,

C = Time specific conductance/observed conductance

= 3 milli mhos.cm^{-1} / K_o millimhos.cm^{-1}

= x (dimensionless)

[**Note:** For most of the conductivity cells, cell constant is between 0.5 to 2.0. The cell before use must be made either dry or be rinsed with the experimental solution]

Experiment - 16B

Determination of the Dissociation Constant, K_a of a Weak Acid, (Say Acetic Acid) at Various Dilutions and hence to Verify Ostwald's Dilution Law Conductometrically

Theory:

The ionization extent of a weak acid (say acetic acid) is very low. In aqueous solution of a weak organic acid let the degree of ionization be α, Ionization equilibrium may then be represented as :

$$HA + H_2O \rightleftharpoons H_3O^+ + A^-$$

At equilibrium: C (1 – α) Cα Cα and the equilibrium constant, k_a, as:

$$K_a = \frac{[H_3O^+][A^-]}{[HA]} = \frac{Ca \times Caa^2.C}{C(1-a)(1-a)}$$

$= \alpha/(1 - \alpha) \,.\, V$ as concentration is inversely proportionate to volume,

Where

C = Concentration of weak acid solution in normality

α = degree of ionization of the weak acid

$= \lambda/\lambda_\infty$

Where, λ = equivalent conductance at a given dilution and

λ_∞ = equivalent conductance at infinite dilution

Conclusion:

Since the value of the dissociation constant, k_a, is nearly constant for the various concentration of the weak acid, (k_a = ... At room temperature) Ostwald's dilution law is verified. From the equation [$k_a = \alpha^2/(1-\alpha).V$] it is clear that as V increases, α (degree of ionization) must increase accordingly so as to maintain the value of k_a constant.

Procedure:

Acetic acid solutions of various dilutions (e.g. 0.5 N, 0.25 N, 0.125 N, 0.0625 N) are prepared in distilled water.

The conductivity cell is washed with distilled water and rinsed with the respective solutions before measuring the conductance of each one of them.

The cell constant C, is generally known from the supplier's manual or determined before hand as described in experiment number 16.1.

The conductivity cell of known cell constant value is then immersed completely in the specified solution and its conductance is determined. Similarly the conductance of other prepared solutions are also calculated.

(*Note:* Sufficient quantity of each solution must be used so that the platinum electrodes are completely immersed into the solution).

Calculation : Temperature of the solution = ...°C (usually room temperature)

: Cell constant C = ... (as determined or supplied)

: λ_∞ = equivalent conductance at infinite dilution

Acid solution (here CH_3COOH)	Observed conductance k_o	True specific conductance $k = k_oC$	Equiv. inductance $\lambda = 1000k/C$	$\alpha = \lambda/\lambda_\infty$	$K = \alpha^2C/(1-\alpha)$
0.5 N	Mmho.cm^{-1}	Millimho.cm^{-1}	Mho.cm^2		
0.25 N					
0.125 N					
0.0625 N					
					Mean K =

Experiment - 16C

Determination of the Solubility of a Sparingly Soluble Salt (AgCl) by Conductivity Method at Room Temperature and hence also KS_p (Solubility Product of AgCl)

Given the known value, λ_∞ of AgCl solution = 138 $Ohm^{-1}.cm^{-1}$; cell constant C

Procedure:

Cell constant is first determined or known. The conductivity cell is washed 3-4 times with distilled water and then immersed in distilled water contained in a beaker and maintained at the specified temperature.

The appropriate range is selected and the conductance of water (k_w) is read. This k_w is the specific conductance of water.

A portion of a dilute KCl solution is taken and to it is added required amount of $AgNO_3$ (silver nitrate solution) when AgCl will get precipitated. The precipitate is separated by filtration and washed several times (7-8 times) with 7-10 mL of distilled water at a time by decantation. To the washed precipitation is added about 50 mL of distilled water with continuous stirring. All these process are required to prepare a saturated solution of AgCl at the temperature of the experiment. The conductance of this solution is then determined (i.e. noted down). This is k_δ. The specific conductance of this solution is k_{AgCl} solution = $k_{(obs.)} \times C$

Data: The specific conductance of water = $k_{water} = k_W$ .... $Ohm^{-1}cm^{-1}$ – Specific conductance of saturated AgCl solution in water = k_{AgCl} solution = $k_{(observed)} \times$ Cell constant $ohm^{-1}.cm^{-1}$

Calculation:

For the saturated solution of AgCl in water, λ is replaced by λ_∞ since AgCl has very low solubility (S) in water and thus,

$$\lambda_{\infty(AgCl)} = 1000k_{AgCl}/S, \text{ Therefore, S(solubility)} = \frac{1000 \times (k_{AgCl\ soln.} - k_{water})}{\lambda_{\infty(AgCl)}} \text{ in g.equi / L}$$

and hence, $K_{Sp(AgCl)}$ i.e. solubility product of AgCl = S^2 $(g.equi.)^2/L$

Experiment - 17

Refractometry

Theory:

The refractive index of a medium with respect to vacuum is given by the equation:

$\mu = \sin i / \sin r$ = Angle of incidence/Angle of refraction

= Velocity of light in vacuum (or air)/velocity of light in the medium

Specific refractivity of a substance is given by $r = (\mu^2 - 1)/(\mu^2 + 2).d$

Where, d = density of the medium

Molar refractivity of the medium is given by the equation:

$$R_M = (\mu^2 - 1)/(\mu^2 + 2).M/d$$

Where, M is the molecular weight of the substance

It is important to remember that molar refractivity R_M is an additive as well as a constitutive property.

Experiment - 17A

Determination of the Concentration of a Supplied Sample (say KCl, NaCl or $BaCl_2$) in Solution by using a Refractometer

Procedure:

The prisms of the Abbe's refractometer are required to be cleaned and dried (by gentle touching with filter paper strips) before every use.

A standard solution of the supplied sample (say KCl or NaCl of 5-6% w/v concentration) is prepared first. From this a series of 5 solutions of differing concentrations are prepared.

A few drops of the experimental sample are placed on the surface of the lower portion of the prism and sandwiched it between the prisms.

The mirror below is adjusted for maximum reflection of light and then viewed through the eye-piece. The position of the prism is adjusted with the help of the knob so that the boundary line between (bright and dark) is in the field of view. If the boundary line is not sharp and is colored (rainbow) it is removed by adjusting the circular disc provided for the purpose. The cross-wire is brought exactly on the boundary i.e. the point of intersection of the cross coincides with the boundary.

The refractive index is read on the scale provided for the purpose. Let it be μ_w for water. If the reading is not 1.333 at around 25°C a correction factor is calculated using the equation : $k = (1.333 \pm \mu_w)$ at the temperature of the experiment and then corrected value of refractive index is then = $\mu_{corrected} = (\mu_o + k)$

Similarly, the refractive indices of each solution of known concentrations and also of the supplied sample solution are noted.

Then a graph of refractive indices μ *vs* concentrations is plotted. It must be straight line from which the concentration of the supplied sample is obtained.

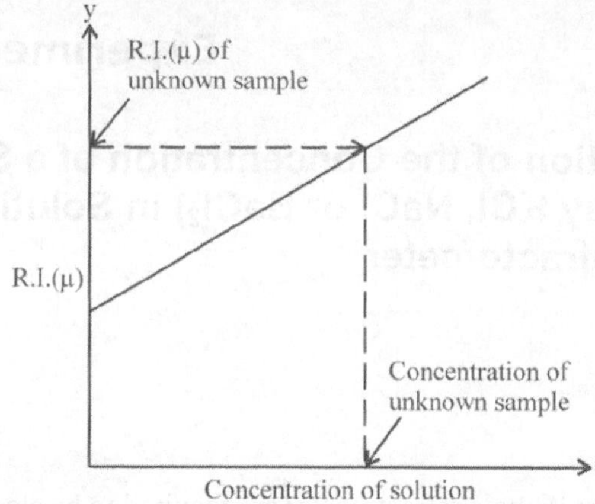

Fig. 17.1 Refractive index (R.I) (μ) Vs. concentration plot.

Experiment - 17B

Determination of the Percent Composition of a Binary Liquid Mixture of Two Liquids using a Refractometer

Given sample A (let it be CCl_4 or any other liquid miscible with the second sample B); Sample B = C_6H_6 as because CCl_4 is miscible with benzene.

D_A = density of the sample A = 1.585 g/mL for CCl_4 at 25°C and d_B = density of the sample B = 0.874 g/mL for C_6H_6 at 25°C

Apparatus: Abbe Refract meter

Procedure:

The prisms of the refract meter is cleaned with alcohol using soft filter strips and dried completely before each use with different liquid(s).

The procedure for using the refract meter is same as described in experiment number 17.1 (i.e. the previous one).

The refractive index (R.I.) of distilled water is first determined. If it is not 1.333 at around 25°C, then correction factor is determined (discussed in the previous experiment 17A). Let it be μ_w (observed) then corrected value will be $\mu = \mu_{obs} + k$, where, $k = (1.333 - \mu_{obs})$

After cleaning and drying process of the prism a few drops of liquid A (CCl_4 in this case) were placed on the lower prism and then closed with the upper one. Since the liquid may evaporate (in case of volatile liquids) it is added with a pipette through the tiny hole at the gap between the two prisms and R.I. reading is noted from the scale. Let it be μ_A observed.

Similarly, the refractive index of the second liquid B(C_6H_6) and also of the mixture containing A and B (i.e. μ_c) are determined.

The density of the mixture d_c is also measured
d = mass/v = [weight of a known volume (V) of the mixture]/V

[**Note:** If μ_{obs} for water is less than 1.333 (i.e. $\mu_{obs} < 1.333$) then positive sign for k (correction factor) is used or vice versa]

Calculation:

If C_A and C_B be the respective per cent concentration of A and B in the mixture, then,

$$r_c = (r_A.C_A)/100 + (r_B.C_B)/100 = (r_A.C_A)/100 + r_B(1 - C_A)/100 \quad .....(1)$$

Substituting the values of r_A, r_B, r_c from the observation as described by equation (1) which is known as Lorentz and Lorenz equation: $r = (\mu^2 - 1)/(\mu^2 + 2).1/d$, where the terms have their respective usual significance and $R_M = (\mu^2 - 1)/(\mu^2 + 2)$. M/D from this equation molar refraction of each liquid can be determined

Result: % by weight of A in the mixture = ……………..%

% by weight of B in the mixture = ……………..%

Precautions:

The prisms should never be touched, cotton or filter paper strips are to be used for drying.

Boundary (black and white) should be made very sharp by adjustment. Special care should be taken while using volatile liquid.

Experiment - 18

Polarimeter

Polarimeter is the instrument that is used to measure optical activity (i.e. Optical rotation) of an optically active substance.
Now what is optical activity?

Ordinary light is a transverse wave motion and the oscillations are at right angles to the direction of propagation of light waves.

When, by some mechanism, all or part of the oscillations in different planes are made to turn from their original planes so as to vibrate in one plane, the light is said to be polarized. Plane polarized light is, therefore, the one which has light vibrations restricted to a single plane only.

By passing light through a polarizing prism, a Nicol Prism, the randomly distributed vibrations of radiation are sorted out so that only those vibrations occurring in a single plane are emitted. Thus, plane polarized light is the one which has light vibrations restricted to a single plane. The velocity of this plane polarized light can become slower or faster as it passes through a medium. This change in velocity results in refraction of the plane polarized light in a particular direction for an optically active substance. A clock-wise rotation, looking into the beam of polarized light, defines a substance that is dextro-rotatory where as anti-clock-wise rotation characterizes a laevo-rotatory one. The dextro-rotatory substance rotates the beam of polarized light to the right, produces an angle of rotation, θ, that is defined as positive, while the laevo-rotatory substance would rotate the beam to the left, has an angle, θ, that is assigned a negative sign.

Molecules having an asymmetry, that is, lacking in symmetry about a single plane is optically active.

The rotatory power of the substance concerned is expressed in terms of specific rotation $[\alpha]_{\lambda}^{t}$, such that

$$[\alpha]_t^l = \theta / 1.d \qquad .....(1)$$

Where, θ is the observed rotation of the polarised beam at t°C caused by l-decimeter (dm) of liquid of density, d, λ is the wave length of the light used.

In the case of a solution of concentration, C, expressed in gram/cm^3; $[\alpha]_\lambda^t = \theta/l.C = 100.\ \theta/l.C$, for 1.0% solution.

The specific rotation is, thus, the rotation produced by a solution containing 1.0g of the substance per centimeter cube (cm^3) when the length of the column through which the light passes is 10 cm (i.e., 1 dm). The specific rotation is a characteristic property of the optically active species.

The molar rotation hs been given as:

$$[\alpha_M]_\lambda^t = M[\infty]_\lambda^t\ /100 \quad .....(2)$$

Analyser is another Nicol's prism placed co-oxially with the polarized and is used to measure the angle of rotation.

Experiment - 18A

Determination of the Specific Rotation of an Optically Active Substance and hence to verify its Purity and also to Determine the Concentration of the given Substance in Solution

Materials: A polarimeter, polarimeter tube (20 cm = 2 dm in length), optically active substance (glucose/sucrose), etc. a source of monochromatic light (usually Na-vapor lamp, yellow color)

Procedure:

From a freshly prepared stock solution of known strength (10% w/v solution) 4 to 5 more solutions of specified concentrations (say, 2.0, 4.0, 5.0, 6.0, 8.0) are prepared by dilution using 50 mL or 100 mL volumetric flasks.

The polarimeter tube is filled with distilled water after first washing and rinsing with it. Care should be taken to see that there is no air bubble in the tube. If a tiny air bubble is there, then it is made to get trapped into centre "bulge" so that it is not in the path of light.

The light source (Sodium lamp, yellow light) is switched on and viewed through the eye-piece and the analyzer screw is rotated to obtain the uniform circle of "minimum light". Adjustment should be such so that the two halves are equally illuminated for minimum intensity. The main scale reading and the vernier scale reading are noted. The reading with distilled water is the "zero reading" of the instrument. The reading is taken when intensity of light on the two halves of the eye-piece is the same i.e. the dark half is equally illuminated as the other half.

The angles of rotation for the prepared solutions of known strength are then determined in the same manner.

Data: Room temperature ....°C, length of the tube = ...

$$\text{Least count}\ (\text{L.C.}) = \frac{\text{Minimum divisions on main scale}}{\text{Number of divisions on vernier scale}\ (\text{dm})}$$

Therefore, Observed Reading = Main scale reading + (vernier scale reading × L.C.)

Solutions % (w/v)	(Observed angle of rotations) (i)	(ii)	(iii)	θ corrected angle	Specific rotation $[\alpha]_{\lambda}^{t}$, = 100θ/L.C.
% (water)					
2.0%					
4.0%					
5.0%					
6.0%					
8.0%					
10.0%					
Unknown solution (x)					Mean $[\infty]_{\lambda}^{t}$, = ...

Calculations:

Since, $[\alpha]_{\lambda}^{l}$,= 100θ/l.C; then θ ∞ C

As $[\infty]_{\lambda}^{t}$, is the specific rotation of the optically active substance at fixed wave length λ and temperature t is a constant, and l, the length of the tube is also constant.

Therefore, plot of θ *vs* C should be a straight line passing through the origin (0,0).

From the straight line graph the conc. of the unknown solution is computed.

Result: The mean specific rotation of the given optically active material; $[\infty]_{\lambda}^{t}$, = ... conc. of the unknown sample solution = ...% w/v

Experiment - 18B

Determination of the Composition of a given Binary Mixture of Two Components in which one is Optically Active

Given: A solid-solid mixture

Apparatus: Polarimeter, polarimeter tube,

Chemicals: An optically active substance (say, sucrose or glucose) an inert material (say, NaCl or KCl)

Procedure:

A. A standard plot of θ *vs* concentration is constructed using different concentrations of the optically active component (supplied, sucrose in this case). At the very outset "zero" of the polarimeter is determined using distilled water. A standardized stock solution (10% w/v) is first prepared and then using this solution four more diluted solutions of pre-fixed concentrations (2.0, 4.0, 6.0 and 8.0% w/v) are prepared by dilution with distilled water in 100 mL volumetric flaks. The angle of rotation (θ) of each solution including that of the stock is determined using polarimeter tube of length 2.0 dm.

   The standard plot of θ *vs* concentration is obtained using the observed data.

B. After accurately weighing 10 g (w) of the supplied sample a 10% w/v solution is prepared and its angle of rotation (θ) is observed using the tube of 2 dm length.

Calculation:

From the standard plot the percent concentration (x) of the optically active substance in solution is computed.

Therefore, 'x' g of component (A) i.e. optically active component is present in 100 mL of the solutions and the rest (100 – x) is the weight of the inert material in % w/v and hence 10x% of active and 10y% = {(10 – x)*100/10} = (100 – 10x) %w/v

Precautions:

Monochromatic light (Na-temp) is to be used only. The tube is required to be rinsed with the given solution in each case.

Mean of at least three readings is recorded. No air bubble should be present in the path of light.

Experiment - 18C

Determination of the Order of Acid-Hydrolysis of Sucrose (or any other Optically Active Substance) at Room Temperature using a Polarimeter

Given: A 15% or 20% w/v solution of sucrose.

Apparatus: Polarimeter and polarimeter tube (2 dm), a monochromatic light source (Sodium lamp usually).

Chemicals: Source, HCl solution (3 N)

Theory:

Sucrose is dextro-rotatory, but its hydrolysis yields glucose and fructose of which the former is dextro-rotatory and the latter is laevo-rotatory. The laevo-rotatory power of fructose being greater than that of glucose the angle of rotation goes on decreasing with time during hydrolysis. The course of reaction can, thus, be studied by measuring the angle of rotation at various time intervals from the start of hydrolysis. The resultant solution at the end becomes laevo-rotatory and this phenomenon of conversion from dextro-side to laevo-rotation is known inversion of cane sugar solution.

$$C_{12}H_{22}O_{11} + H_{20} \xrightarrow[\text{HCl (glucose) fructose} \atop \text{(+ve)} \quad \text{(−ve)}]{[H^+]} C_6H_{12}O_6 + C_6H_{12}O_6$$

Procedure:

The "zero" of the instrument using distilled water is to be determined (or checked) first. It is the polarimeter reading of the distilled water.

The prepared (or supplied) sample of a specified sample solution (usually 15% or 20% w/v) of the optically active sample is diluted with 2 N HCl (or 3.0 N, 4.0 N). HCl solution to get the resultant 10% sugar solution and the time of mixing noted. This is θ_o at time to. The polarimeter tube (usually of 2.0 dm in length) is then filled up with the resultant solution (taking care that there is no air gap in the tube) and the angle of rotation at pre-determined time-intervals (say at t = 3,6,10,15,20,30,40 and 60 minutes from the start of the reaction at room temperature.

The angle of rotation at t = 0 may be obtained by using a 10% w/v sample solution diluted with distilled water and determining the angle of rotation θ_o.

The infinity reading, θ_∞, is obtained by allowing the reaction mixture to "stand" for 24 hrs. or more after which period reading is taken.

Data obtained: Water bath (or room temp.) = ... °C

θ_o at zero time.

θ_∞ after completion of the reaction i.e. the infinity reading.

θ_t = angle of rotations at 't' times.

Then, a (initial concentration) = $(\theta_\infty - \theta_o)$ and (a – x) (i.e. concentration at the specified time interval) = $(\theta_\infty - \theta_t)$

Time in minute	θ_t (a – x) = $(\theta_\infty - \theta_t)$, log (a – x)
3	
6	
10	
15	
20	
30	
40	
60	
etc..............	

The k (specific rate constant) = 2.303/t log [a/(a – x)].min^{-1}. Then mean k value is calculated. Graphical representation of log (a-x) *vs* t would yield a straight line indicating that acid-hydrolysis of sucrose solution is a first order reaction. Then from the slope reading k is calculated.

Result: k = ... min^{-1}

The two results are then compared.

Experiment - 19

Experiment on Partition Co-efficient

Theory:

If a solute is added to a binary system consisting of two immiscible liquids contained in a stoppered bottle and if the solute is soluble in both the liquids, the solute, then, gets partitioned (or distributed) between the two solvents and the equilibrium condition is reached when the chemical potential of the solute in the two solvents is the same. At this equilibrium point the ratio of concentration of the solute in the two solvents is a constant at a given temperature. This equilibrium constant is called the partition co-efficient (P) or the distribution co-efficient, k_d, of the solute between the two solvents.

Mathematically,

$$P \text{ (or } k_d) = C_{\text{Organic phase}} / C_{\text{aqeous phase}} \qquad .....(1)$$

This condition is valid only when the solute goes into solution as molecular dispersion without undergoing either association in organic phase or dissociation in the aqueous phase.

In case of association, say, n molecules of the solute associate in the solvent (organic, O) and there is no dissociation of the solute in the aqueous phase, the above equation does not hold good and the modified equation.

$$K_d = \frac{n\sqrt{C_{or.}}}{C_{aq.}} \text{ or } \frac{C_{or.}^{1/n}}{C_{aq.}} \qquad .....(2)$$

Or $\log K_d = 1/n \log C_{or.} - \log C_{aq.}$ Or $(1/n)\log C_{or.} = \log K_d + \log C_{aq.}$ is only applicable.

If there is dissociation of the solute in the aqueous phase and no association in the organic phase the equation to be applied is as :

$$K_d = C_{or.} / C_{aq.}(1-\infty) \qquad .....(3)$$

Where, ∞, is the degree of dissociation (or ionization) of the solute in the aqueous phase.

In case of association and dissociation taking place in the two solvents, the modified equation is:

$$K_d = \frac{C_{or.}^{\ 1/n}}{C_{aq.}(1-\infty)} \text{ or } \frac{n\sqrt{C_{or.}}}{C_{aq.}(1-\infty)}$$

It is to be noted that the partition co-efficient of a solute between two given solvents depends on temperature but it is independent of the amount of solute or solvent used. At the time of determining partition coefficient care must be taken to avoid saturation point of the solute in either phase, otherwise, deviation will occur.

Experiment - 19A

Determination of the Partition Coefficient of Benzoic Acid between Water and Benzene

Materials and Methods

Materials: A 5.0% w/v solution of benzoic acid in benzene. 4 stoppered bottles (100 mL capacity), 0.1 N NaOH and 0.01 N NaOH solutions standardized with accurately weighed and prepared solution of oxalic acid in water.

Method: The four stopepred bottles are cleaned and dried. In the four containers labeled A, B, C and D four different solutions of varying concentrations are prepared as follows:

In (A) 30 mL of benzoic a solution in benzene (5% w/v) is taken and then 30 mL of benzoic acid solution + 40 mL of water in (C) 15 mL of 5.0% benzoic acid solution + 45 mL distilled water and in (D) 10 mL of the benzoic acid solution + 50 mL distilled water.

The stoppred bottles are shaken for 30 minutes and allowed to stand for 20 minutes by which time the two layers would separate into two distinct layers slowing a sharp interface. It is required to be ensured that equilibrium has been attained during the resting period.

10 mL of the aqueous solution (lower denser layer) is pipette out into a conical flask (or a beaker) containing some 20 mL of water and then titrated against 0.01N NaOH solution using phenolphthalein as the indicator. End point : Colorless – pink. (Precaution: While pipetting out from the lower layer the pipette and should be closed with the thumb so that no solution from the upper (or lighter) layer can enter into the pipette. Otherwise, mixing will take place).

Then 2 mL of the solution from the upper benzene layer is pipette out using a dry pipette and is added to 20 mL of water taken in a beaker. It is the titrated with 0.1N NaOH solution using phenolphthalein as the indicator: End point – pink, (Precaution: While pipetting out from the upper layer care is to be taken to avoid smoking from the interface. The tip of the pipette should be held fixed at the middle point of the upper layer. Benzoic acid being a surface active agent maximum concentration would be at the interface).

Calculation: Using the formula:

Volume of NaOH solution consumed in each case × Normality of NaOH solution used × milli equivalent weight of the substance (benzoic acid in this case) = weight of the substance in grams.

Then using equation $K = C_{org.}/C_{aq.}$ or $K = \sqrt{C_{org.}}/C_{aq.}$

Partition co-efficient of the material is determined. The equation which yields nearly constant values of K is the right equation.

Alternately or simultaneously K (distribution constant) may also be obtained by plotting $\log C_{aq.}$ *vs* $\log C_{org.}$, when slope = 1/n, n (number of association) is then computed.

Result: K = ………….. at ………..°C and if $C_{aq.}/\sqrt{C_{org}}$ is nearly constant in each case benzoic acid exists as a dimer (i.e. n = 2) in benzene.

Experiment - 19B

Determination of the Distribution Coefficient of Salicylic Acid between Water and Benzene

Materials: Sodium salicylate benzene, volumetric flasks (100 mL), pipette, test tube, ferric nitrate, distilled water.

Procedure: Students will work in pairs.

A-1: An accurately prepared solution of sodium salicylate (40 mg per mL) will be required for each pair of students. Accurately 5.00 mL of this solution is pipette out and delivered into a 100 mL volumetric flask and q.s. with distilled water. (Be very peruse, since this solution will represent your standard solution). The standard solution just prepared represents a concentration of sodium salicylate equal to 2.00 mg per mL.

The following solutions are then accurately prepared :

Solution (1)	5 mL of the standard solution / 100 mL water
Solution (2)	10 mL of the standard solution / 100 mL water
Solution (3)	15 mL of the standard solution / 100 mL water
Solution (4)	20 mL of the standard solution / 100 mL water
Solution (5)	25 mL of the standard solution / 100 mL water

A-2: The quantitative determination of sodium salicylate is based on the estimation of the purple color produced by the addition of ferric nitrate solution to the sample. The purple color produced will be quantitatively with a spectrophotometer at 525 (millimicron, mμ) read against a blank.

Six test tubes are then arranged in the following manner :

Test Tube (1)	1 mL of the solution no. 1 + 2 mL of ferric nitrate solution + 5 mL of distilled water.
Test Tube (2)	1 mL of solution no. 2 + 2 mL of ferric nitrate solution + 5 mL distilled water
Test Tube (3)	1 mL of solution 3 + 2 mL of $Fe(NO_3)_3$ solution + 5 mL distilled water
Test Tube (4)	1 mL of solution 4 + 2 mL $Fe(NO_3)_3$ + 5 mL distilled water

Test Tube (5) 1 mL of solution 5 + 2 mL $Fe(NO_3)$ + 5 mL distilled water

Test Tube (6) 6 mL of distilled water + 2 mL $Fe(NO_3)_3$ solution

This solution of Test tube 6 is the blank for the experiment.

The obserbance of each of the above 5 solutions is determined and absorbance (A) is plotted *vs* mg. of Na-salicylate / mL i.e., A *vs* concentration (in mg/mL). This "Beer plot" should yield a straight line with an intercept of zero.

The partition co-efficient of salicylic acid between water and benzene is determined by placing exactly 25 mL of the solution of concentration 2.00 mg mL^{-1} in a 125 mL glass stoppered bottle and exactly 25 mL of benzene is added.

The bottle is stoppered, shaken vigorously and intermittently for 20 minutes and allowed to stand for some time till the two phase separate out completely – 10 mL of the aqueous phase solution is then withdrawn. (Core should be taken to avoid entry of any benzene phase from the upper benzene layer into the pipette while withdrawing aqueous phase solution from the bottom layer. This is achieved by closing the open end of the pipette with the thumb before hand). The salicylic acid concentration is estimated by developing color on adding of 2.00 mL $Fe(NO_3)_3$ solution as previously described.

The experiment is required to be done in duplicate.

The concentration of salicylic acid content in the benzene phase is calculated by difference. The partition coefficient (K_d) as defined:

$$K_d = \frac{C_{Benzene}}{C_{Water}}$$ is then computed.

Experiment - 19C

Determination of the Partition (Distribution Equilibrium) Constant of Iodine between Water and Carbon Tetrachloride (CCl_4) or Chloroform ($CHCl_3$)

Materials: A 8% w/v (approximate) solution of iodine in CCl_4 or Chloroform ($CHCl_3$), CCl_4 or $CHCl_3$ (which one is supplied), 0.1 N, $Na_2S_2O_3$ and very dilute 0.005 N $Na_2S_2O_3$, separating funnels etc.

Procedure:

1. In four different separating funnels four solutions of varying concentration are prepared as follows :
   (a) 40 mL of I_2 solution in CCl_4 + 40 mL distilled water
   (b) 30 mL of I_2 solution in CCl_4 + 10 mL CCl_4 + 40 mL water
   (c) 25 mL of I_2 solution in CCl_4 + 15 mL CCl_4 + 40 mL water
   (d) 20 mL of I_2 solution in CCl_4 + 20 mL CCl_4 + 40 mL water

   The funnels are shaken intermittently for about 30 minutes allowing time for iodine to get distributed between the two solvents and for distribution equilibrium to reach equilibrium point. The funnels are then allowed to stand for 10-15 minutes till the two solvents separate out forming a distinct interface. The lower (i.e. denser) CCl_4 layers are then drained out of the funnel into four different (marked, a, b, c and d) dry Stoppard bottles. The aqueous layers remains in the separating funnels.
2. 10 mL of the aqueous layer is pipette out using a dry pipette and it is titrated against 0.005 N $Na_2S_2O_3$ solution using starch solution as the indicator.

   End point is violet to colorless. The procedure is followed in each of the four CCl_4 layer samples.
3. Next, 5 mL of the CCL_4 layer is pipette into a container (a conical flask) containing 0.1g (approx.) of KI in 10-15 mL water and it is titrated against 0.1 N $Na_2S_2O_3$ using the starch solution as the indicator near the end point (i.e. when a faint iodine color still persists). End point will be reached when CCl_4 layer as well as the aqueous layer in the titration flask is colorless. Constant shaking of the titration flask is

needed during titration. Pipette used must be dry. The procedure is followed for the remaining samples too.

Data obtained: Temperature of the experiment......................°C

Sample No.	$T_{aq.}$	$T_{org.}$	$N_{aq.} \approx C_{aq.}$	$N_{org.} \approx C_{org.}$	$K = C_{aq.} / C_{org}$
1					
2					
3					
4					

$T_{aq.}$ = mL of 0.005 N $Na_2S_2O_3$ consumed per 10 mL of aqueous layer.

$T_{org.}$ = mL of 0.1 N $Na_2S_2O_3$ consumed per 5 mL of organic layer

$N_{aq.}$ = Normality of the aqueous layer (calculated after titration)

$N_{org.}$ = Normality of the organic layer (as calculated after titration)

$C_{aq.}$ = Concentrated in g/L of aqueous layer

$C_{org.}$ = Concentrated in g/L of the CCl_4 layer

K = partition co-efficient of T_2 between water and CCL_4 at room temperature..........°C

[For calculation of $N_{aq.}$ and $N_{org.}$ the equation to be used is $V_1N_1 = V_2 \times N_2$]

If $K = C_{aq.} / C_{org.}$ is not constant in the series then the equation $K = C_{aq.}/n\sqrt{C_{org.}} = C_{aq}/C_{org.}^{1/n}$ is to be applied to determine the value of n (the association number) Or graphically, $\log C_{aq.} = \log K + 1/n \log C_{org.}$, by plotting log $C_{aq.}$ against log $C_{org.}$ n is calculated from the slope.

For any convenient point on the line log $C_{aq.}$ corresponding log $C_{org.}$ is considered. Substituting these values and the value of the slope in the final equation. $\text{Log } C_{aq.} = 1/n \log C_{org.} + \log K$ the value of K is obtained.

[If n = 1, iodine ha its normal molecular weight in both the solvents (aqueous and organic). Entry of aqueous layer into the pipette while pipetting out organic layer must be avoided].

Experiment - 20

Adsorption at a Solid-liquid Interface

Theory:

Solids have the property of holding molecules at their surfaces, particularly if the solids are finely divided and porous. The amount of solute adsorbed from solution by a unit weight of solid increases with the quantity of solute in solution, i.e. with the increase of solute concentration in solution. The equilibrium between the dissolved solute and that adsorbed also depends on the nature of the solvent and the temperature. Generally the less soluble the solute or the lower the temperature, the greater the extent of adsorption.

The relationship between the amount adsorbed and concentration may be represented by a number of equations. The simplest is an empirical relationship known as the Freundlich equation:

$x/m = K.C^{1/n}$; where, x = weight of the solute adsorbed by m grams of adsorbent,

C = concentration of the solution, and 1/n (i.e. n) and K are constants. By taking logarithms of this equation we get :

$$\text{Log } x/m = 1/n \log C + \log K$$

As plot of (log x/m) *vs* (log C) is a straight line and the constants may be evaluated from the slope (1/n i.e. n) and the intercept (log K).

A theoretical equation related to the Freundlich equation is then derived by Langmuir :

$$x / m = \frac{K_1 K_2 C}{1 + K_1 C}$$

Where, x, m and C are the same as previously mentioned and where K_1 and K_2 are constants. Rearrangement of the Langmuir equation yields :

$$C/(x/m) = (1/K_1K_2) + (C/K_2)$$

Now, using this equation, when C/(x/m) is plotted versus C a linear plot should occur with slope equal to $1/K_2$ and the intercept = $1/(K_1K_2)$. The significance of K_1 and K_2 (i.e. adsorption coefficient and adsorption capacity terms need discussion in the class).

Each pair of students will be given a solid which is water insoluble, commonly used in pharmaceutical products. These may include starch, talc, kaolin, calcium carbonate, titanium dioxide (all in their activated states) and also activated charcoal. The affinity of these solids for an anionic dye may be measured in the laboratory experiments. The dye, with the following structure, is typical of the certified dyes used in pharmaceuticals.

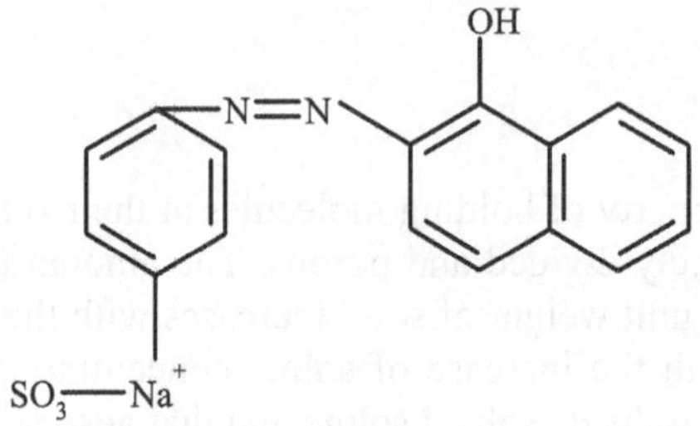

Procedure:

50 mL each of 0.05%, 0.025%, 0.01%, 0.005% and 0.0025% dye in water (all prepared from a standard stock solution by dilutions) are added to 2.00 g of assigned solid. This weight of the solid (the adsorbent) should be known to the nearest 0.10 g. The mixture is allowed to sit, with occasional stirring, for one hour to insure equilibrium. After that 1 mL of supernatant solutions is removed from the two solutions of highest concentrations, using a glass wool plug. This is then put into a 100 mL volumetric flask and brought to volume with water. 5 mL are then removed from each of the remaining three containers and then added to a 50 mL volumetric flask and brought to volume by dilution with water. These diluted samples are measured colorimetrically. While waiting for equilibrium, the five original solutions must be measured colorimetrically in the same manner as described above.

For each of the 5 solutions, computed the following quantities, the equilibrium concentration in mgs/L, $C_{eq.}$ the number of mg of dye adsorbed, x; the ratio of this weight to that of the solid, x/m. Three plots, x/m *vs* $C_{eq.}$, log x/m *vs* log $C_{eq.}$ and $C_{eq.}/(x/m)$ *vs* $C_{eq.}$ are to be plotted. The, the respective constants of the Freundlich and Langmuir equations are to be calculated.

In order to compare the adsorbing properties of the various solids (Pharmaceutical), the values for x/m and $C_{eq.}$ should be obtained from other fellow students. Then x/m *vs* $C_{eq.}$ for these various solids are to be plotted for comparing the degree of adsorption on each solid.

Experiment - 20A

Determination of the Specific Surface Area (area/g) of a given Powder (Activated Charcoal as an Example)

Materials: Stoppard bottles, 0.50 N acetic acid, 0.10 N standard NaOH solutions.

Procedure:

The normality of the given or prepared 0.50 N acetic acid solution is first determined by titrating with 0.10 N standardized sodium hydroxide solutions using phenolphthalein indicator. Let the normality be No. End point: Colorless – pink.

Acetic acid solutions of different concentrations (normalities) are prepared in different bottles dried completely beforehand as follows:

Stoppard bottles N_o	1	2	3	4	5
mL of standardized solution acetic acid	50	40	30	20	10
mL of distilled water	0	10	20	30	40
Concentration in g equi/L (normality)	N_o	4/5 N_o	3/5 N_o	2/5 N_o	1/5 N_o

[*Note:* Normality of the prepared and standardized solution of acetic acid should be as near 0.5N as possible]

All the experiments are performed at room temperature.

Then, 1.0 g of the activated charcoal (weighed accurately) is added to each of the 5 bottles, shaken for nearly 40 minutes (by swirling occasionally, not continuously) for adsorption equilibrium to be attained during the period.

Each of the above mentioned solutions is then filtered using dry filter paper into fine different dry conical flasks and the normality of each filtered solution is determined by titrating 10 mL of the each filtered solution against standard 0.1 N NaOH solution using the same phenolphthalein solution as the indicator.

Calculations:

10 mL of the stock acetic acid solution = ...T mL of 0.1 N NaOH

N_o = Normality of the given acetic acid solution;
N_1 = Initial normality,
N_2 = Normality of acetic acid solution after adsorption.
C_e = Equlibrium concentration of acetic acid solution (stock) = $N_1.M$ g/L

Where,

M = Molecular weight of acetic acid = 60 = equivalent of acetic acid
x = Amount of acetic acid adsorbed per 50 mL of the solution
= $(N_1 - N_2)/1000 \times E \times 50$; where, N_1 and N_2 have the usual significance,
E = equivalent weight of acetic acid = 60 (Adsorbate) and
m = Mass of the adsorbent (here activated charcoal) in g and
x/m = Amount of adsorbate (acetic acid) adsorbed per gram of adsorbent (charcoal)

The graphs of x/m *vs* C_e and log of x/m *vs* log $C_{eq.}$ are drawn. For graphical representation of the Langmuir isotherm the equation to be applied is :

$C_e/(x/m) = (1/K_1K_2) + C_e/K_2$; where, K_1 = adsorption co-efficient

K_2 = monolayer capcity, a constant quantity = mass of the adsorbate adsorbed per gram of adsorbent to form a monolayer covering the whole surface area till monolayer formation process is complete, or in other words it is also known as saturation concentration (ym) a constant specific of an adsorbate-adsorbent system.

Then, plotting $C_e/(x/m)$ *vs* C_e the slope of the straight line $1/K_2$, (or 1/ym) is obtained from which K_2 (or ym) can be calculated i.e. ym or K_2 = 1/slope and hence the specific surface area of charcoal (in this case) is given by :

S (specific surface area) = (ym/M) × N × A;
where,

M = Molecular weight of acetic acid = 60
N = Avogadro's number = $6.023 \times 10^{23} \approx 6 \times 10^{23}$
A = cross sectional area of acetic acid/molecule = 16×10^{-16} cm^2 per molecule

Result: Specific surface area of charcoal = ...Cm^2/g

Precautions:

Dry filter papers, dry funnels, dry beakers are required to be used.

Acetic acid solutions are to be standardized with standard NaOH solution. Time period for the attainment of adsorption equilibrium is important before filtration.

Experiment - 20B

Verification of Freundlich's Adsorption Isotherm for the Adsorbate (Oxalic Acid/Acetic Acid/ Benzene Acid) and the Adsorbent (Activated Charcoal/any other Inert Adsorbent of Pharmaceutical Interest

Materials: Stoppard bottles, constant temperature batch at room temperature, oxalic acid solution 0.5 N, 0.1 N NaOH solutions (standardized before hand).

Procedure:

As in the previous experiment.

Observation:

As in the previous experiment.

Only difference is that in this case 0.5 N Oxalic acids is being used instead of 0.5 N acetic acid.

Calculations and Graphical Presentation

Freundlich's Adsorption Equation is given by the equation:

$x/m = K.C_e^{1/n}$, where K and n are constants depending on the nature of adsorbent and adsorbate.

Therefore, plot of log x/m *vs* log C_e would yield a straight line yielding the values of constants n and K from the slope (= 1/n) and from the intercept on the y-axis = log K.

Experiment - 21

Hydrophile - Lipophile Balance (HLB)

Theory

It is the amphiphilic nature of surface active agents (i.e. surfactants) that causes them to be absorbed at the interfaces, whether there are liquid-gas or liquid-liquid interfaces. Thus, in an aqueous dispersion of amyl alcohol, the polar alcoholic group is able to associate with the water molecules. The non-polar portion is ejected out, however, because the adhesive forces it can develop with water are small in comparison to the cohesive forces between adjacent water molecules. As a result, the amphilic is adsorbed at the interface.

For the amphilic to be concentrated at the interface, it must be balanced with the proper amount of water and oil-soluble groups. If the molecule is two hydrophilic, it migrates into the body of the aqueous phase and remains there without exerting any effect at the interface. Likewise if it is too lipophilic, it gets dissolved completely in the oil phase and little appears at the interface.

Griffin devised an arbitrary scale of values to serve as a measure of the hydrophilic-lipophilic balance (HLB) of SAA'S; higher the HLB value higher is the hydrophilicity and vice versa.

The equations used are:

The HLB of a non-ionic surfactant whose only hydrophilic portion is poly oxy ethylene is calculated by using the formula: HLB = E/5; where E is the percentage by weight of ethylene oxide.

A member of polyhydric alcohol fatty acid esters, such as glyceryl monostearate, can be estimated by using the formula: HLB = 20 (1 – S/A) where S = saponification number of the ester and A = acid number of the fatty acid.

HLB plays an important role in formulations such as in the preparation of o/w or w/o type of emulsion, anti-foaming agent characterization, suspension preparation etc.

To determine the HLB value of a given Ester:

Apparatuses: Water bath, round bottom flasks, condenser, burette, pipette, conical flasks, etc.

Chemicals: A given ester (may be glyceryl monostearate) 0.1 N NaOH, 0.5 N HCl (both standardized before hand, i.e. exact concentration i.e. normality must be known) 0.5 N alcoholic KOH.

Procedure:

It is carried out in two parts:

A. To determine the saponification value of the ester :

An accurately weighed sample (0.5 g) of the given ester is taken is a round bottom flask and to it is added 15 mL of the 0.5 N alcoholic KOH solution. It is heated on a boiling water bath with a reflux condenser fitted at the end of the RB flask neck for 45-50 minutes. The equation for this hydrolysis is:

$$\text{R-COOR}^{1} + \underset{\text{(alcoholic)}}{\text{KOH}} \longrightarrow \text{R}^{1}\text{OH} + \text{RCOOK}$$

The solution is cooled to room temperature and the whole quantity is titrated using 0.5N HCl solution using phenolphthalein as indicator. Let the titre value be V_1 mL of 0.5N HCl.

A blank experiment is also conducted simultaneously under the same experimental conditions using 15 mL of alcoholic. KOH solution, refluxing for 45-50 min. cooling to room temperature and titrating the whole quantity against standardized 0.5N HCl solutions. Let the titre reading be V_2 mL of the same 0.5N HCl.

B. To measure the acid value of the ester :

An accurately weighed W g (around 0.5g) of the stearate sample is taken in a conical flask, dissolved in 10 mL ethyl alcohol + 10 mL ether (warmed if necessary on a water bath. Caution: Alcohol and ether are highly inflammable) The whole of the sample is then titrated against 0.1 N NaOH solution using the phenolphthalein indicator (end point pink).

Let the titre reading be V_3 mL of 0.1 N NaOH.

Calculations: Saponification value is the number of milligrams of KOH required to neutralize completely the acid obtained by saponification of 1.0 g of the sample (ester).

Saponofication Value: Equivalent wt of KOH = 56g

Quantity of the acid formed by alkaline hydrolysis of Wg (0.50 g) of the ester.

$= (V_2 - V_1)$ mL of 0.5 N HCl

$= (V_2 - V_1)$ mL of 0.5 N KOH

As 1000 mL of 1 N KOH ≡ 56000 mg of KOH

Therefore, $(V_2 - V_1)$ mL of 0.5 N KOH ≡ $56(V_2\text{-}V_1)$ x 0.5 mg of KOH per Wg sample

$\equiv 28(V_2 - V_1)$ mg per Wg sample

Therefore, Saponification value $S = 28(V_2 - V_1)/W$

C. Acid value "A" is defined as the number of milligrams of KOH required to neutralize free acid present in 1.0g of the sample.

Now, Wg of the sample ≡ V_3 mL of 0.1 N NaOH

Therefore, 1.0 g of the sample ≡ (V_3/w) mL of 0.1 N NaOH

As 1.0 N NaOH solution ≡ 1000 mL of 1 N KOH ≡ 56 × 1000 mg KOH

Therefore, (V_3/w) mL of 0.1 N KOH = 5.6 (V_3/w) mg of KOH ≡ "A" the acid value

HLB Calculation: The HLB = 20(1-S/A), thus, substituting the values of S and A in the equation, HLB value is obtained.

Result: The saponification value, "S" =

The acid value, "A" =

The HLB of glyceryl monostearate =

Experiment - 22

On Colloidal Dispersions

Reference: Dutta S.K. – Principles of Physical Pharmacy and Biophysical Chemistry, Chapt.:18. Martin - Physical Pharmacy; Chapt: 18

Colloid state is a particular state of matter or substance. A colloidal system is always a heterogeneous two-phase system. Finely divided particles of any substance with diameters lying between 10 A^{o} - 2000 A^{o} dispersed in any medium constitute what is termed a colloidal system, colloidal dispersion or simply a colloid.

The material with the particle size in the colloidal range (1-200 mμ) is said to be in the colloidal state. The colloidal sols or colloidal dispersions are intermediate between true solutions and coarse suspensions.

Sols are colloidal systems in which a solid is dispersed in a liquid and therefore, are sub-divided into two classes: (a) Lyophilic sols (solvent loving) (b) Lyophobic sols (solvent-repelling).

Lyophilic sols are those in which substances, like proteins, starch, gelatin, polysaccharides such as acacia, synthetic polymers, soaps etc. pass readily into colloidal state whenever mixed with a suitable solvent. Such colloids have strong interactions with dispersion medium and thus, in contrast to the lyophobic sols, are almost in true solution, but because of their macromolecular nature their solutions exhibit colloidal properties. Stabilization is due to salvation and also to the possession of charged ionic groupings on the molecule. Such systems can be coagulated and precipitated by various means but can usually be returned to their colloidal state.

Lyophobic Collids on the other hand, are those in which the dispersed phase has no attraction for or interaction with the external dispersion medium (i.e. solvent). The colloidal nature of such substances results from an extremely fine state of subdivision of the material. Such systems are stabilized by the presence of electrical charges on the suspended particles. Neutralization of such charges results in a coagulation of the system which is irreversible. Example: Gold-sol.

$Fe(OH)_3$ sol; and sol of sulfur in water.

This experiment is designed to illustrate methods for preparing some cols, the nature of their stabilization mechanism and factors influencing the stability.

Procedure:

1. **Preparation of Sols**
   (a) ***Preparation of a sol by hydrolysis:*** Gradually add 50 mL of a 2% (w/v) ferric chloride ($FeCl_3$) solution to 150 mL of boiling water. A colloidal solution (or sol) of $Fe(OH)_3$ is formed (SAVE).
   (b) ***Preparation of a sol by condensation:*** 0.5g of sulfur (approximately) is placed in a small conical flask containing 25 mL of alcohol and the mixture is shaken for several minutes. The suspension is filtered and the filtrate collected in a clean dry beaker.
   2.0 mL of the filtrate is pipette out and poured into 25.0 mL of water with mixing (SAVE).
   (c) ***Preparation of a sol by reduction:*** To 50 mL of distilled water is added 2.0 mL of 0.1N silver nitrate ($AgNO_3$) solution and 1.0 mL of 1% (w/v) tannic acid solution. The mixture is heated to 70°C-80°C and then 1.0 mL of a 1.0% sodium carbonate (Na_2CO_3) solutions is added with through stirring (SAVE).
   (d) ***Preparation of a lyophilic sol:*** 4 g of powdered gelatin is added to 50 mL of water. After 20 minutes 75 mL of water is added and the mixture is heated on a water-batch at 60°C-70°C until all of the gelatin is dissolved. After allowing to cool the volume of the system is made 200 mL by the addition of warm water. (SAVE).

2. **Properties of Sols**
   (a) A small portion of each of the various sols prepared is filtered through ordinary filter paper. Any changes, if observed, is to be recorded.
   (b) The filtrates are held, one by one, in front of a strong beam of light. Any observations need to be explained.

   The experimental observation is done also with filtered distilled water for comparison.

3. **Effects of Electrolytes**

   4.0 M solution of NaCl and a 0.002M solution of Na_2SO_4 are prepared. From each of these two a series of 10 mL portions of diluted solutions are prepared by mixing in test tubes 2, 3, 5, 7, 9 mL electrolyte solute on and 8, 7, 5, 3, 1 mL of distilled water.

Added to each of these solutions 10 mL of $Fe(OH)_3$ solution, mixed well and allowed to stand for an hour. At the end of this time interval it is to be seen in which cases precipitation has occurred and then the molar concentrations of Cl^- ions and SO_4^{2-} ion necessary to produce precipitation are recorded. The experiment is repeated with 10 mL of the gelatin solution using Na_2SO_4 solution only.

4. **Effect of dehydration on lyophilic colloidal stability**

   5 mL of gelatin solution are added to 1, 2, 5, 10 and 15 mL of ethyl alcohol and any changes recorded.

5. **Protective colloidal action**

   As previously described, the concentration of SO_4^{2-} ion required to precipitate 10 mL of $Fe(OH)_3$ sol is determined. To each dilution is added 2 mL water in lesser amount which is replaced by adding 2 mL of gelatin solution instead. Observations need to be recorded.

Experiment - 23

Suspensions

Reference: Dutta S.K., Principles of Physical Pharmacy & Biophysical Chemistry, Chapt.18, Page – 744

A suspension is a coarse dispersion of insoluble solid particles having diameter greater than 0.01 μm in a liquid medium which is usually water or an aqueous based vehicle. Suspensions are biphonic heterogeneous systems and are of much importance in pharmacy and medicine.

Procedure:

Properties of wetting agents and hydrophobic powder:

(a) A piece of raw cotton is placed on the surface of a beaker of water; a 1% aerosol O.T. solution is then added drop wise. What happened to the cotton? Why? The experiment is to be repeated using Tween 80 and the results compared.

(b) In a prescription bottle, 1 g of sulphur and 4 g of charcoal are taken and 100 mL of water is added, shaken well and is observed.

Then after adding 10 mL of each surfactant solution the resultant charges with each surfactant solution added is noted. Observations before and after the addition of these surfactants are compared.

Experiment - 23A

Sedimentation Rate

Two 100 mL of 10% aqueous suspensions of light and heavy MgO to be prepared in two graduated cylinders, thoroughly shaken or stirred with a glass rod until the particles are uniformly dispersed. The two suspensions are then allowed to settle and then height, h, of the clear zone is measured from time to time. A plot of height, h, in cm *vs* time in seconds is drawn in each case. From the initial slope of the line the velocity of sedimentation is determined. The process is to be repeated three times and average value from slopes determined.

The experiment is repeated using CCl_4 (Carbon tetra-chloride) as the medium ($n \approx 0.01$ poise is considered).

Applying Stokes equation

$$v = \frac{h}{t} = \frac{[2r^2 (d_s - d_o)g]}{9n_o} = \frac{[d_p^2 (d_s - d_o)g]}{18n_o}$$

$$= \sqrt{(18n_o h)/(d_s - d_o)gt}$$

To the data the average diameter of the particles is computed. Is there agreement between the data obtained in both solvents ? Which v is [dp the rate of settling (sedimentation), h, is the distance of fall in time t, d_p, is the mean diameter of the particles based on the velocity of sedimentation, d_s, is the density of the particles and d_o that of the dispersion medium, and n_o is the viscosity of the medium] The equation holds good only for spheres falling freely without hindrance and at a constant rate. The particles must not be aggregated or clumped together in the suspension since such clumps would fall more rapidly than the individual particles, and erroneous results would be obtained. The proper deflocculating agent must be found for each sample that will keep the particles free and separate as they fall through the medium.

For Stokes' Law to apply, a further requirement is that the flow of dispersion medium around the particle as it sediments is laminar or streamline. In other words, the rate of sedimentation of a particle must not be so rapid that turbulence is set up, since this in turn, will affect the result. Whether the flow is turbulent or laminar is indicated by Reynolds number,

Re, (dimensionless) which is defined as : $R_e = (v.d_p.d_o)/n_o$ in which symbols have the usual significance.

According to Heywood, Stokes' Law cannot be used if R_e is greater than 0.2, since turbulence would appear at and above this value.

Rearranging the $R_e = (v.d_p.d_o)/n_o$ and combining it with Stokes equation we get:

$$V = (R_e.n_o)/(d_p.d_o) = [d_p^2(d_s - d_o)g]/18n_o \text{ and thus,}$$

$$d_p^3 = (18n_o.R_e.n_o^2)/(d_s - d_o).g.d_o$$

Under a given set of density and viscosity conditions, the above equation allows calculation of the maximum particle diameter, d_p, whose sedimentation rate will be governed by Stokes' Law, that is when R_e will not exceed 0.2.

Using a modified equation known as Carman Kozeny equation: (To be discussed in class): $V = [d_p^2(d_s - d_o)g]/18n_o \times e^3/(1 - e)$; where e = the porosity of the particles and other terms are the "Stokes" variables, density, diameter and viscosity, the calculations are to be repeated for verifying the validity of the results obtained.

[Porosities of the light and heavy MgO may be determined by the practical methods as practiced in the laboratory]

Experiment - 23B

Sedimentation Rate in the Presence of Surfactants and Electrolytes

Procedure

The samples containing heavy MgO in water and in CCl_4 (prepared in the above described experiment) are used in this experiment. The two samples are allowed to stand undisturbed for 12-24 hours. The following suspensions:

(a) 0.1% aerosol O.T

(b) 0.25% aerosol O.T

(c) 0.1 M NaCl and let them also to settle in graduated

Cylinders are prepared, the rate of sedimentation in each case is followed and the observations compared with that in water.

These samples are allowed to stand for 12-24 hours. When measuring the final settling volume results may be recorded as volume in mL of settled particles per gram of solid. In order to allow the cylinders to be used during the next laboratory session – the suspensions are transferred into labeled prescription bottles and set aside until next practical class date. At that time each sample is decanted and a drop of each sample is observed under a microscope fitted with micrometer to estimate the size of particles. Is there any correlation between the size of the particles and the liquid medium used? Report your results.

Experiment - 23C

Relationship between Suspension Caking and Zeta Potential

Procedure:

A 100 mL suspension of 2% bismuth subnitrate in 2% acacia solution is prepared. Likewise in each sample of 2% acacia suspension (prepared) contained in separate bottles 0.4 mM, 4.0 mM, 40 mM and 400 mM $AlCl_3$ solution is added; these samples are allowed to sit for weak. At that time the suspension is checked for possible difference in the case of dispensing them by shaking the bottle.

Correlate your results with the electrical nature of each suspension

Experiment - 23D

Determination of the Concentration Range which the Electrolyte (say, $AlCl_3$) Acts as a Deflocculating Agent for Kaolin Suspension (say of 10%)

Materials required: 10 glass-stoppered tubes of about 30 mL capacity, kaolin, aluminum chloride ($AlCl_3.6H_2O$) 100 mL of 5% (w/v) solution of $AlCl_3$ in distilled water.

Procedure:

A stock solution of 5% (w/v) $AlCl_3,6H_2O$ is first prepared, and using this solution aqueous solutions of varying concentrations ranging from 0% to 2.0% (w/v) are prepared by dilution with distilled water to make the final volume of each solution to 25 mL. Then 2.5 g of kaolin is added into each solutions. The test tubes are stoppered, shaken well and allowed to stand in a vertical position undisturbed. Observations, are made at various time intervals to ascertain the nature of sediment, whether particles are loosely packed or compact sediment is formed. Data are arranged in tabular form:

Observations:

Table 23.1 Observations

Test Tube	Vol. of 5% $AlCl_3$ added (mL)	Water added to make the Vol. 25 mL	Conc. of prepared $AlCl_3$ (% w/v)	Wt. of Kaolin taken (g)
1	0	25	0	2.5 g in each Test Tube
2	0.05	24.95	0.01	
3	0.10	24.90	0.02	
4	0.20	24.80	0.04	
5	0.50	24.50	0.10	
6	1.00	24.00	0.20	
7	2.00	23.00	0.40	
8	2.50	22.50	0.50	
9	3.00	22.00	0.60	
10	10.00	15.00	2.00	

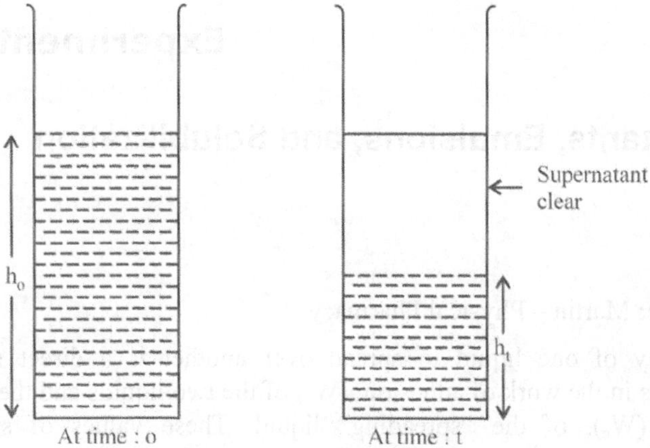

Fig. 23.1 Sedimentation behaviors of Kaolin Suspension after setting.

Nature of the supernatant and nature of the sediment, and also whether the particles are loosely packed or forming compact sediment are to be ascertained and reported (in your laboratory notebook).

Result:

The flocculated suspensions are: (lower sides of $AlCl_3$ suspension)

The deflocculated suspensions are: (at higher concentration above…..)

Experiment - 24

Surfactants, Emulsions, and Solubilization

Reference: Martin – Physical Pharmacy

The ability of one liquid to spread over another is a direct result of differences in the work of adhesion. (W_a) of the two liquids and the work of cohesion (W_e), of the "spreading" liquid. These values of spreading coefficient, S, can be calculated by using the equation :

$S = W_a - W_e = \gamma_1 - (\gamma_1 + \gamma_{1,2})$; where, S = Spreading coefficient.

γ_1 = Surface tension of the sub-layer liquid

γ_2 = Surface tension of the spreading liquid

$\gamma_{1,2}$ = Interfacial tension existing at the interface between the two liquids (To be determined by a convenient surface tension measurement method, say Drop-Count Method or Capillary rise method).

Spreading will occur when S-value is positive, that means the surface tension of the sub-layer liquid is greater than the sum of the surface tension of the spreading liquid and the interfacial tension of the spreading liquid and the interfacial tension between the two liquids.

If $(\gamma_2 + \gamma_{1,2}) > \gamma$, the spreading liquid will form globules or a floating long and will fail to spread over the surface.

The ability to spread therefore, is an indication of some "affinity" between immiscible liquids, or in thermodynamic terms, the free energy at the interface is reduced when spreading takes place.

One would summarise that such "affinity" can only arise when chemical groups, capable of interaction are present in both of the substances. Likewise, this implies that orientation of molecules at the interface must occur.

Procedure:

A 250 mL beaker is thoroughly cleaned with soap/cleaning mixture and water then rinsed with water. About 100 mL of water (distilled/tap water/de-ionized water) is taken in the beaker, and some lycopodium powder sprinkled lightly onto the surface. After waiting for the powder to stop moving, a drop or two of the liquid (supplied) placed onto the surface in the centre of the beaker.

Observe and report what occurs with the following liquids:

(a) A mineral oil and / or

(b) Oleic acid

Indicate qualitatively the relative ability of these substances to spread on water. How do these observations compare with literature values of initial spreading co-efficient?

Emulsions:

1. 80 mL of water and 20 mL of mineral are taken in a prescription bottle. This is to be repeated with Oleic acid. The bottles are shaken vigorously for 2-3 minutes and allowed to stand. The time required for each system to separate completely into two phase are to be compared. How does this compare with their spreading behaviors (i.e. properties)?

   Now, using the same systems, the liquid system is passed through a hand homogenizer which allows more force to break droplets down to a fine size. The time needed for separation to occur is then noted.

   Does passage through a homogenizer aid in the formation of emulsions? If yes, why? (Save for future comparison).
2. 10-12 g of mineral oil + 1.5 g of span 80 + 3.5 g of Tween 80 + 35 mL of water are taken in a stoppered prescription bottle and shaken vigorously. Observations to be compared with those of the first experiment.

   The preparation is passed through a hand homogenizer and the results compared (Save).
3. To a mixture of 30 g of mineral oil + 3 g of Arlacel 83 in a stoppered prescription bottle is added 30 mL (≡ 30 g) of water very slowly with vigorous agitation. It is, again, passed through a homogenizer if necessary.

[**Note:** The homogenizer must be washed thoroughly after each solution is passed through it. If oil globules are left behind in the homogenizer, they may crack the emulsion on the next passage through the homogenizer].

Determination of Emulsion Type

A. Electrical Conductivity Method:

This method is based upon the fact that an aqueous solution is a much better conductor of electricity than is oil. Thus the electrical resistance of an oil-in-water (o/w) emulsion would be much less than that of water-in-oil (w/o) type.

The emulsion to be tested is placed in a beaker and the platinum electrodes attached to a conductivity bridge, are dipped into the preparation.

Resistance is recorded. This procedure is then followed with both mineral oil emulsions.

Apparatus and chemicals: Conductivity meter, conductivity cell, emulsion No.1 and emulsion No.2; KCl solid.

Emulsion 1: 25 mL water + 1 mL coconut oil, vigorously stirred with a glass rod. This is o/w type

Emulsion 2: 25 mL coconut oil + 2-3 mL distilled water vigorously stirred. This is w/o type.

Given: Specific conductance of 0.02 N KCl solution = 3 mmho. cm^{-1}

Procedure: Firstly, the conductivity meter needs to be "standardized". The conductivity cell is washed with deionized water, dried gently with a piece of filter paper strips, dipped in the 0.02 N KCl solution, Knobs adjusted for cell constant. The "standardize" Knob is then adjusted to read the conductance of the solution as 3 milli mhos. The conductivity meter is thus, "standardize" top read the correct conductance value.

The electrodes are washed and then conductance of de-ionized (or distilled) water is then read after selecting the appropriate range. The conductance value of water (K_w) is obtained.

The same method is followed to get the conductance values for Emulsion 1 (k_1) and Emulsion 2 (k_2).

To each of the two emulsions 10 mg of solid KCl is added and mixed thoroughly. The conductance values K_1^1 and K_2^1 are then obtained. It is observed that there is sudden increase in the conductance is the first case (i.e. Emulsion No.1) and in the second case is of a lesser value (nearly zero).

Result: Emulsion 1 is of o/w type and
Emulsion 2 is of w/o type

B. Dilution Method

A drop or two of the emulsion placed onto a water surface. If it tends to thin out over water, or if mixes readily with the water, the emulsion is of the oil-in-water type. If the emulsion drop does not tend to mix or to spread, it must a w/o emulsion.

C. Dye Method

A drop of oil soluble dye solution is added to a portion of the emulsion. If the oil is the continuous phase the color will spread throughout the body of emulsion. If the oil is the dispersed phase the individual oil droplets become colored upon stirring the dye into the emulsion.

If water soluble dye solution is used reverse will be the observation.

Observe the emulsions under a microscope.

Compatibility of surface active agents:

100 mL of 1% aqueous solutions of the following surfactants prepared and kept stored in stoppard prescription bottles.

(a) Sodium lauryl sulphate
(b) Benzal konium chloride
(c) Tween 80
(d) Aerosol O.T.

A] 5 mL of a 1% $CaCl_2$ solution is added to 5 mL of each of the solution.

B] To each of the above solutions 1 mL of benzal-konium chloride added.

From your observations, indicate which of above mentioned solution (s) could not be used in products requiring preservation by benzal konium chloride.

C] Added 5 mL of O^- in HCl solution to each of the above mentioned solutions. Observations?

Reasons

Phase-volume ratio: 50 mL of a 10% solution of Arlacal C dissolved in vegetable oil is taken in a 250 mL beaker, water in 5 mL increments is added with rapid manual stirring and changes in the apparent viscosity are noted after each addition.

Why does the viscosity increase with the addition of water? At what point does the emulsion crack?

Cloud point determination: The water-soluble polyoxyethylene non-ionics are less soluble in hot than in cold water. These surfactants are thought to dissolve by the association of water molecules with the other linkages. At higher temperatures, this association is partially destroyed, causing the surfactant to become less soluble.

The temperature at which the solubility of the surfactant is greatly reduced is marked by a change from a clear to a turbid solution, and is known as the cloud point. The larger the ratio of ethylene oxide units to hydrophobe, the more water soluble the compound becomes. The higher the H.L.B., higher will be the temperature at which, the cloud point occurs.

Solubilization:

A. Micelle Formation

A 0.005% w/v solution of benzopurpurin 4B, a dye (or % any other suitable dye) is first prepared. Using this solution a series of Tween 20 solutions of the following concentrations are prepared.

0.001%, 0.002%, 0.004%, 0.008%, 0.01%, 0.02%, 0.04%, 0.08%, 0.1%, 0.5%

A solution of only 0.005% dye in water is also prepared which will be the blank in this experiment.

Next, the surface tension of each of the prepared solution is measured. After measuring the surface tension of these solutions, the absorbance of each solution at the wave length of 530 mμ is measured. The simple dye solution being the blank the differences in absorbance are noted.

Would you observe any abrupt changes in the surface tension and absorbance pattern at the same concentration? If yes, why? Explain.

B. The following formulations are to be prepared and solubilization pattern observed.

A	B	C	
Lavender Oil	1/2 %	1/2%	1/2%
Tween 20	4%	6%	10%
Water	95%	93%	89%
(50 g of each)			

	A	B
Coal Tar	1g	1g
Tween 20	2g	--
Water q.s. ad	50 mL	50 mL

Tween 20 is to be added to the coal tar in a glass mortar and triturated well, water added slowly with constant trituration.

	A	B
Benzoic Tincrture	2 mL	2 mL
Glycerin	15 mL	15 mL
Tween 20	5 mL	---
Water q.s. ad,	60 mL	65 mL

Firstly, the benzoic tincture is to be mixed with the Tween 20; Glycerin mixed with water is gradually added to the first dispersion with constant stirring.

The differences to be observed. Give your comment on the findings.

Experiment - 25

Rheology
(i.e. Flow Properties)

1. **Effect of Salvation on Viscosity:**

   To each of three small beakers containing 1.0g of Na-alginate, added 20 mL of water to the first beaker, 20 mL of glycerin to the second beaker and 20 mL. of alcohol to the third one, stirred well. The relative solution of the sodium alginate by each of the solvents is to be noted by observing the aggregation of particles as well as the consistency of the particles.

   Next, 10 mL of the alcohol slurry of Na-alginate is added to 40 mL of water and stirred well. By what mechanism does the alcohol assist in dispersing the alginate in water? Give your comments from your acquired knowledge.

2. **Effect of Temperature on Viscosity:**

   A 250 mL of a 1.0% solution of methyl cellulose, 400 is to be prepared in the following manner:

   (a) 150 mL of water contained in a calibrated 250 mL beaker is allowed to boil.

   (b) After boiling has commenced, heat source is removed and the methyl cellulose content slowly added with constant stirring. When the methyl cellulose is completely dispersed, ice chips are slowly added with constant stirring; the final volume of the preparation should be 250 mL.

   (c) 250 mL of a 1.0% solution of methyl cellulose 4000 is also to be prepared in a similar manner.

   (d) The use of hot water in the preparation of methyl cellulose is compared with the use of alcohol in the preparation of Na-alginate.

   (e) Heat 100 mL of methyl cellulose 400 preparation and report your observations.

3. **Effect of pH on Viscosity:**

   Carbapol 934 is a water soluble resin used as a suspending and emulsifying agent. The viscosity of Cabapol 934 dispersions is dependent on pH of the dispersion medium.

A 20 mL sample of a 0.50% carbapol 934 is to be titrated with 1.0mL increments of 0.1 N KOH (standardized beforehand). 80,000

The transitions that occur are to be noted down.

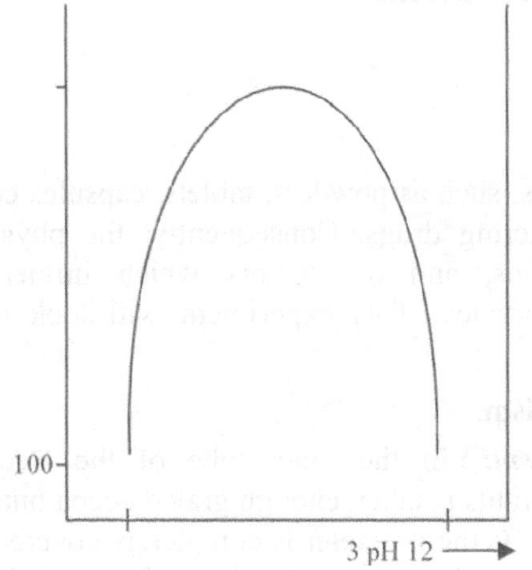

Fig. 25.1

4. Viscosity Measurement:

(a) Instructions for the use of the Stormer Viscometer should be carefully reviewed as described in the manual with each instrument.

Water is placed in the thermostat bath of the viscometer to maintain some control of temperature.

With a stopwatch, the time required for 100 revolution is measured using a 505 w/v glycerin-water mixture,. Since this mixture is Newtonian the velocity, v, in revolution per second is determined for 3 driving weights, w, 100 g, 125 g, and 150 g.

Since: $\acute{\eta} = K_s.(w/v)$; where, $\acute{\eta}$ = viscosity in poise and K_s is a constant, one may determine K_s, from known values of $\acute{\eta}$ and corresponding w/v. Is this value of K_s constant for this system?

(b) Measure also the viscosity of the following preparations using at least 4 weights:

1. Methyl cellulose, 400
2. Methyl cellulose, 4000
3. Bentonite magma which has been vigorously agitated just prior to measurement (using only 1 weight).
4. Bentonite magma which has been allowed to remain undisturbed in the instrument a few moments prior to measurement (using the same weight).

Experiment - 26

Properties of Solids

Solid dosage forms, such as powders, tablets, capsules constitute the major mode of administering drugs. Consequently, the physical and chemical properties of solids, and the factors which influence them, are of considerable importance. This experiment will look at certain relevant properties as:

(a) Polymorphism

Polymorphism: In the inner tube of the Beckmann Molecular weight apparatus is taken enough grated cocoa butter so that the bulb of a 0°C-100°C thermometer is completely covered. This tube is then placed into the air-jacket and in turn, this assembly is placed into a beaker of water. The temperature of the bath is carefully raised so that the sample thermometer never reads higher than 34°C-35°C. The cocoa butter should completely melt at this temperature. When only a liquid is present, immediately place the tube without the air-jacket, into an ice-bath. Stirring should be continued as much as possible during the procedure. When the temperature has reached 0°C and solidification is complete, the sample tube is taken out of the ice-bath, placed in the air with the air-jacket in its position and temperature rise is noted every 30 seconds until liquefaction begins. After reaching 20°C the whole assembly is placed in a water bath for slow warming.

At what temperature does it melt?

Comments: This entire procedure, but this time heating the cocoa butter to 45°C until complete liquefaction occurs. The sample is allowed to remain at 45°C for at least half-an hour.

Compare the melting points of cocoa-butter under both sets of conditions. Is there any difference in melting points noted? If so why?

(b) Bulk Density:

True density, void-space volume and porosity constitute properties, which along with particle size distribution, must be known before attempting to formulate any solid dosage form.

If one places, a given weight of solid in a graduated cylinder, the weight of the sample (w) divided by the volume (V_B) occupied, will give the bulk density of the sample.

If the particles of powder (granule) has no spaces between them, this density will be equal to the true density of the sample.

The porosity, e, of a powder (or granule) is the relative volume of void spaces between the particles, V_v to the bulk volume of the sample, V_B. Since, V_v is the difference between V_B and the volume occupied by the particles themselves, V_p.

$$E\ (\text{porosity}) = (V_B - V_P)/V_B \qquad \text{.....(1)}$$

$$= 1 - (V_P/V_B) = 1 - \frac{\text{wt / true density}}{\text{wt / bulk density}} \qquad \text{.....(2)}$$

or

$$e = 1 - \frac{\text{bulk density}}{\text{true density}} \qquad \text{.....(3)}$$

Experiment - 26A

Determination of the Bulk Density of a given Powdered (or granular) Sample

Procedure:

In a tared beaker 100 g of drug granules are taken and weighed to get the weight, W_g These are then placed in a 100 mL or 250 mL graduated cylinder, and tapped gently until a minimum volume is reached. The volume (V mL) occupied by the granules is noted and recorded.

The bulk density of the given granule sample = W/V (g/mL)

Note: For a given sample of powder / granule

Bulk volume > Granule volume > True volume i.e.
Bulk density < Granule density < True density

Light and heavy magnesium oxide (about 25 g of each) may also be used for determining bulk density and porosity.

Experiment - 26B

Determination of the True Density of a given Powdered (or granular) Sample

For non-porous sample (also non-wetting) a sample of sand may be used (particle diameter of about 1 to 2 mm).

In a 100 mL volumetric flask distilled water is poured filling it up to the 100 mL mark. Then 25 mL of water is pipette out with the help of a 25 mL capacity pipette.

A certain amount of the sample (say 50 g or 100 g) is weighed (w_1 g) and from the weighed sample particles are slowly and carefully added to the flask when the water level would start rising. The process of adding is stopped when the level rises back to the 100 mL mark. The remaining powder or granules sample is the weighed again (this is, say, w_2 g).

Therefore, weight of the sample added to the flask = $(w_1 - w_2)$ g

Volume of the sample added = 25 mL

Calculation:

Assuming that the sample is non-porous and non-wetting by nature, the true density would be:

$$D_{true} = (w_1 = w_2) \text{ g/25 mL} = \text{..............g/mL}$$

Note: The liquid used for the expt. Should not wet the particles.

Experiment – 27

Particle Size Distribution Techniques

A particle size specification is considered as an important guidance to the drug substances and it is critical to drug product performance (i.e., dissolution, solubility, bioavailability, content uniformity, stability, or product appearance) or drug product manufacturability (i.e. processability). Other than these from a pharmaceutical perspective, the most critical parameter for an inhalation product is usually the aerodynamic particle size distribution of the emitted aerosol. For solid oral dosage forms, the impact of particle sizes of pharmaceutical powders on drug product manufacturability is of noteworthy importance due to the fact that the majority of the unit operations for manufacturing of solid oral dosage forms are associated to manipulation of the particle sizes of pharmaceutical powders. For instance, granulation and coating are related to particle size enlargement, while milling and grinding are related to particle size reduction. Screening and sieving are related to separation of particles with different sizes. Mixing and blending are correlated to the blend of particles of different components where size differences among these components have a large impact on blend homogeneity. Therefore, understanding the impact of particle sizes of pharmaceutical powders on manufacturing processes is significant for each drug application. The particle size of powders is standardized according to the IP descriptive terms, such as, very fine, fine, moderately coarse, coarse, and very coarse.

The purpose of particle size analysis is to obtain quantitative data on the mean size, particle size distribution and shape of the compounds to be used in pharmaceutical formulation. The particle size analysis is also necessary to reassure the quality of the final dosage forms and drug delivery systems. In addition, now a days technique have been developed for incorporating particle size instrumentation into the process monitoring and control including automated production units. Thus, to enable selection of the most appropriate or optimal sizing technique, cross-correlation between different techniques may be required.

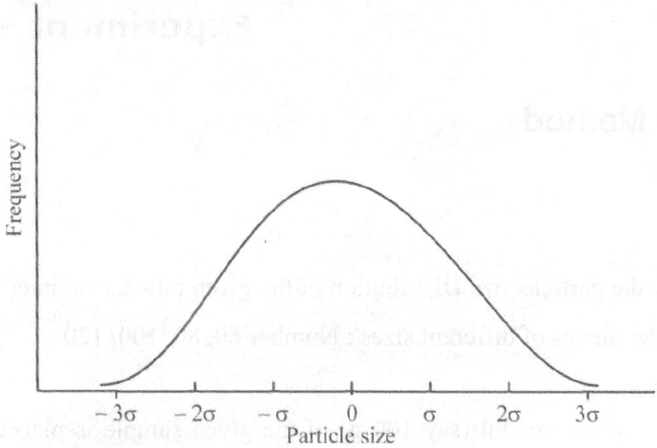

Fig. 27.1 Normal frequency distribution curve (bell shapes).

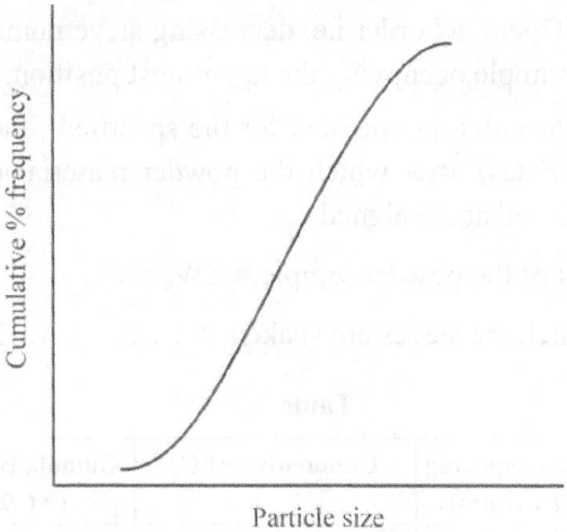

Fig. 27.2 Cumulative % frequency Vs. particle size plot.

Experiment - 27A

Sieve Method

To study the particle-size Distribution of the given powder sample.

Materials: Sieves of different sizes : Number 60, 80, 100, 120

Method:

1. A weighed amount (say 100 g) of the given sample is placed on the sieve of the maximum openings (Lowest sieve number).
2. All the sieves are arranged on the shaker one above the other in increasing "Opening" order i.e. decreasing sieve number; the one with the powder sample occupying the uppermost position.
3. The shaker machine in operated for the specified time period (say for 10 to 15 minutes) after which the powder material retained by each sieve is collected and weighed.

   Total weight of the powder sample = ΣW_n

   Time for which the sieves are shaken = ... Minute.

Table

Sr. No	Sieve No	Sieve opening (......µm)	Cumulative wt C_g	Cumulative % frequency (= $C/\Sigma W_n \times 100$)
1			w_1	-
2			$w_1 + w_2$	-
3			$w_1 + w_2 + w_3$	-
4			$w_1 + w_2 + w_3 + w_4$	-
5			$w_1 + w_2 + w_3 + w_4 + w_5$	-

Graph: Two graphs are to be plotted (1) % frequency (i.e. wt %) *vs* diameter, d, in µm (i.e. sieve opening) and (2) cumulative % frequency *vs* d (µm).

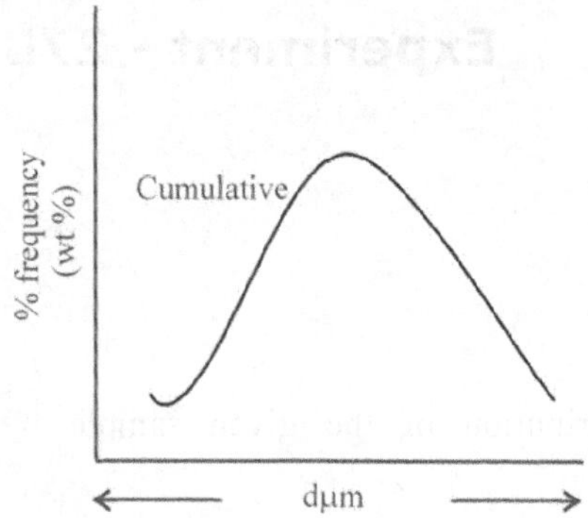

Fig. 27A1 Frequency distribution curve.

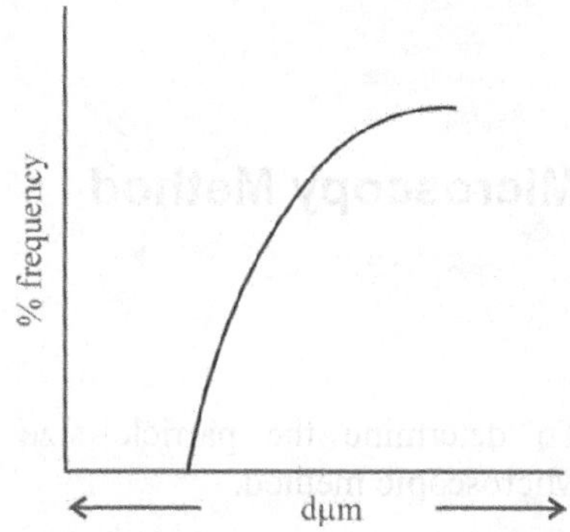

Fig. 27A2 Cumulative % frequency.

Experiment - 27B

Microscopy Method

To determine the particle size distribution of the given sample by Microscopic method.

Materials: Microscope, microscope stage micrometer, water insoluble powder (say Mgo powder)

Procedure:

1 The least count "L" of the stage micrometer is noted first; then, the number of diversions, n_1, of the stage micrometer that coincide with the eye-piece micrometer divisions, n_2 are determined. The 1(one) division of the eye-piece micrometer = $(n_1 \times L)/n_2$

2 A dilute suspension of the given sample in distilled water is prepared and a drop of the suspension is placed on a glass slide and observed the particles under the microscope with the calibrated eye-piece micrometer.

3 The average particle size is evaluated by taking mean of the length and breadth of the particle (since most of the particles are not spherical). At least 100 particles are to be counted for average size measurement.

Note: Usually 1 division of stage micrometer = 0.01 mm i.e. "L" = 0.01 mm

Calculations:

Let a = length of the particle in micron

b = breadth of the particle in micron

Then, Mean size = (a+b)/2

Table Calculations

Size-range (micron)	Mean size d, in micron	d^2	d^3	Tally mark	Frequency	% frequency $n/\Sigma n \times 100$	Cumulative frequency %	nd	nd^2	nd^3
0-0.5	0.25				n_1	f_1	f_1			
0.5 – 1.0	0.75				n_2	f_2	$f_1 + f_2$			
1.0 – 1.5	1.25				n_3	f_3	$f_1 + f_2 + f_3$			
1.5 – 2.0	1.75				n_4	f_4	↓			
2.0 – 2.5	2.25				n_5	f_5	↓			
and so on					etc	etc	↓			
							etc.			
1 micron = 10^{-4} cm = 10^{-6} m					Σn = Total no. of particles			Σnd	Σnd^2	Σnd^3

Graphs: Same as in the previous experiment

Length-number mean diameter = $\Sigma nd/\Sigma n$ = ... micron

Surface-number mean, $d_s = \sqrt{\Sigma(nd^2)/\Sigma n}$ = ... micron

Volume-number micron, $d_y = 3\sqrt{\Sigma(nd^2)/\Sigma n}$ = ... micron

Results:

1. The graph of % frequency *vs* particle size, d indicates that the given powder is polydispersed.
2. The graph of cumulative % frequency *vs* d, is sigmoidal indicating the polydispersed nature of the supplied sample.
3. The statistical diameters are:
   (i) Length number mean diameter, d = ... micron
   (ii) Surface number mean diameter, d_s = ..., micron
   (iii) Volume number mean diameter, d_v = ... micron

Precautions:

1. The eye-piece micrometer is required to be calibrated with a stage micrometer.
2. Dilute suspension to be used to avoid aggregate.

Experiment - 27C

Anderson Pipette Method

The determination of particle-size distribution of a given suspension [also termed as Sedimentation method to construct the frequency (weight) distribution curve].

Materials: Andereason pipette, An aqueous suspension evaporating dish, Distilled water (viscosity of which is ή = 0.008 poise at room temperature), etc.

Note: If Andreason pipette is not available, a 100 mL measuring cylinder of uniform diameter may be used and a 10 mL pipette may be used to withdraw the suspension sample.

Procedure:

The Andreason pipette is placed on a flat surface and the given suspension is poured into it up to the uppermost mark, A, on it. The pipette is inserted in its position; the set-up is shaken well and then kept standing in a vertical position without disturbing it. This starting time (t = 0) is noted.

At t = 10, 20, 30, 40, 50, 60 seconds a fixed volume (10 mL) of the sample is withdrawn each time with the help of the pipette and allowed it to run onto a previously weighed evaporating dish using the two-way stop-cock. The height "h" is the level noted after every withdrawal at t = 0, 10, 20 ………….. etc.

The withdrawn samples collected on each evaporating dish are then heated to complete dryness and weighed to get the weight of the dry solid mass on each dish.

Results: Room Temperature…………….°C

Table 27C1 Observation

Time (Sec.)	0	10	20	30	40	50	60	70	80	90	100
m_2	-										
m_1	-										
W= (m_2-m_1)	-	W_1	W_2	W_3	W_4	W_5	W_6	W_7	W_8	W_9	W_{10}

Significance:

m_2 = Weight of the dish + dried suspension mass

m_1 = Weight of the dish only

w = Weight of the solid mass (dispersed phase)

"h" = height of the suspension column above the lower tip of the pipette.

P_o = density of water (medium) = ………..g/mL

P = density of particles = …………g/mL

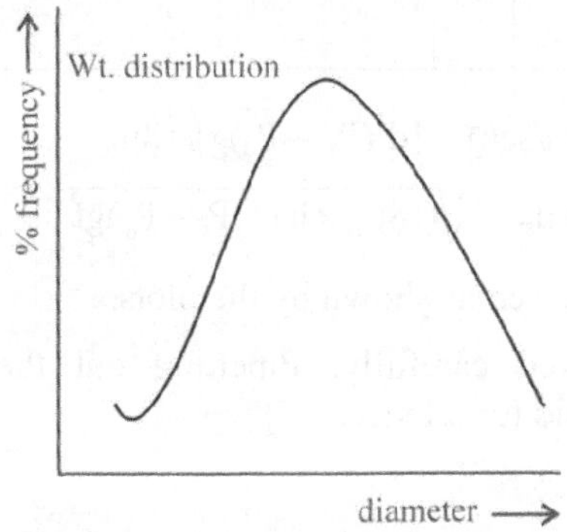

Fig. 27C1 Frequency distribution curve.

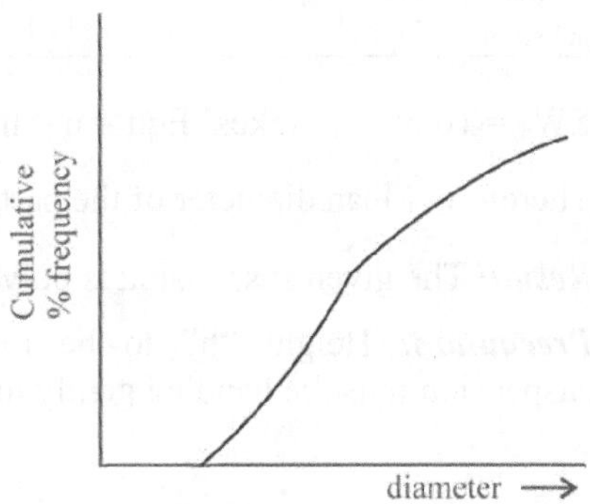

Fig. 27C2 Cumulative % frequency.

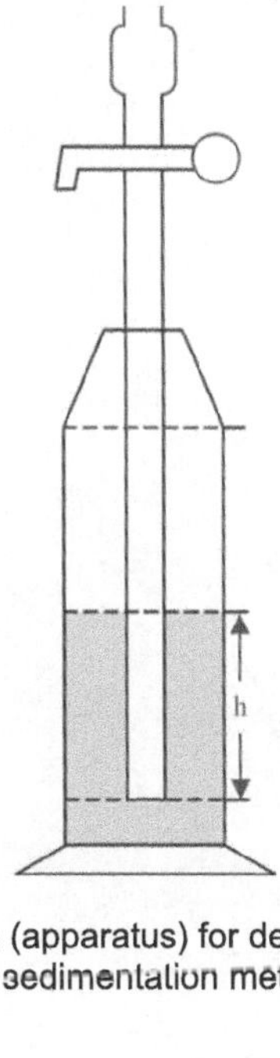

Fig. 27C3 Anderson Pipette (apparatus) for determining particle Size by gravity sedimentation method.

Table 27C2

Time C	"h" Height (cm)	W	Wt % = $[W/\Sigma W_n] \times 100$	u = h/t (cm/sec)	d_{st} (cm)	Cumulative wt; C	Cumulative % frequency $(C/\Sigma W_n) \times 100$
0		-					
10		w_1				w_1	
20		w_2				$w_1 + w_2$	
30		w_3				$w_1 + w_2 + w_3$	
45		w_4					
60		w_5					
70		w_6					
80		w_7					
and so on							

ΣW_n = Total wt; Stokes' Eqn = u = h/t (cm/sec) = $[d^2(P_s - P_o)g]/18\mu_o$

Therefore, Mean diameter of the particles $d_{st} = \sqrt{(18\mu_o \times h)/(P_s - P_o)gt}$

Result: The given suspension is polydispersed as shown by the plots.

Precaution: Height "h" to be measured carefully; Pipetting out the suspension must be handled gently to avoid turbulence.

Experiment - 28

Thixpotropy Measurement

To study the thixotropic behavior of a given or prepared non-Newtonian system using Brookfield/Stormen Viscometer.

Materials: Brookfield viscometer with difference spindles Acacia gel.

Thixotropy may be defined as "an isothermal and comparatively slow recovery on standing of a material of the consistency lost through shearing". Thixotropy is applied only to shear-thinning systems. The most apparent characteristic of a thixotropic system is the "hysteresis loop" formed by the up- and down-curves of the rheogram. This area of hysteresis loop has been proposed as a measure of thixotropic breakdown.

Procedure:

100 mL of acacia gel in distilled water is prepared in a 200 mL beaker (weighed amount x_g/100 mL). The "spindle" is inserted into the gel and it is attached to the Brookfield viscometer taking care that the spindle is just at the surface of the gel mass.

The motor is put into operation by selecting speed of 5 r.p.m. The rotating scale which locks the pointer on the scale is raised. After the specified time period the operation is stopped and the angle of rotation "θ" noted (with practice one can stop the motor so that the pointer is viewed through the window scale). By releasing the lever the disc is lowered.

The readings "θ" for various speeds on the spindles, such as, 5, 10, 20, 30, 40, 50 and 100 r.p.m. are taken. After taking the last (highest) speed reading the spindle is kept rotating for 1 to 2 minutes, and then the readings "θ" for speeds 100, 50, 40, 20, 10, 5 are again noted to construct the "down curve".

Result: Acacia gel = % w/v in D water

Room Temperature = °C

Spindle speed (r.p.m.)	Angle of rotation "θ"
5	:
10	:
20	:
40	:
50	:
100	:

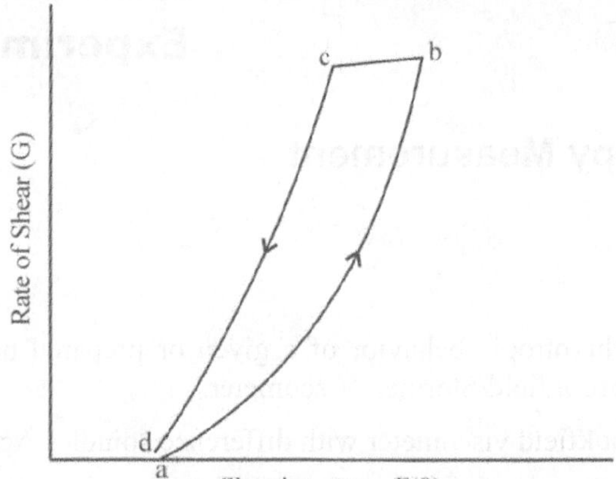

Fig. 28.1 Plastic system exhibiting thixotropic behavior.

(*Note:* The speed of the spindle is proportioned to the rate of shear and the angle "θ" by which the pointer logs behind is proportional to shear stress).

Conclusion: The down curve is shifted to the left of the up-curve and have the given system is thixotropic in nature and thus shows pointer thixotropy. Hence, the system is a non-Newtonian one.

Precautions:

1. The Brookfield viscometer should be handled with care following the instructions of the manual supplied with the instrument. Care must also be exercised while fixing and removing the spindle.
2. Before using the material some practice is needed as to how the pointer is arrested and rotations of speeds stopped for various speeds so that the pointer could be viewed through the "window".

Experiment - 29

Measurement of Angle of Repose

The frictional forces in a loose powder can be measured by the angle of repose, φ. This is the maximum angle possible between the surface of a pile of powder and the horizontal plane. If more material is added to the pile, it slides down the sides until the mutual friction of the particles producing a surface at an angle φ, is in equilibrium with the gravitational force. The tangent of the angle of repose is equal to the coefficient of friction μ between the particles.

$\tan \phi = \mu$, Hence, the rougher and more irregular the surface of the particles, the higher will be the repose angle.

To improve flow characteristics, materials termed glidants are needed for mixing with granular powder.

Procedure:

To study the effect of particle size on the angle of repose the following materials are needed:

A glass funnel, granules or powdered samples of varying sizes (e.g. $CaCO_3$, MgO powder)

Sieves of varying meshes are arranged one above the other in the order of increasing pore size. 500 g of the powder sample (granules) is placed over the uppermost sieve, shaken for 10 minutes on a mechanical shaker. The granules or powder samples of different size ranges are collected.

A glass funnel is clamped in a vertical position above a piece of white paper, a given sample size powder is slowly added into the funnel which gets collected on the paper sheet forming a cone of powder. The circular base of the powder cone is marked with a pencil. The height of the powder cone, h, is then measured.

Data collected are to be arranged in a Table form for sieve no. IP to be consulted:

Powder sample		**Av. Particle size mm**	**d mm**	**h cm**	**r cm**	**Φ**	**tan φ = h/r**
Passed through	Retained						

Where, h = height of the cone, d = diameter of the cone

R = d/2 (radius), φ = Angle of repose

Result:

The nature of the plot of φ *vs* particle size indicates that the angle of repose depends on the particle size.

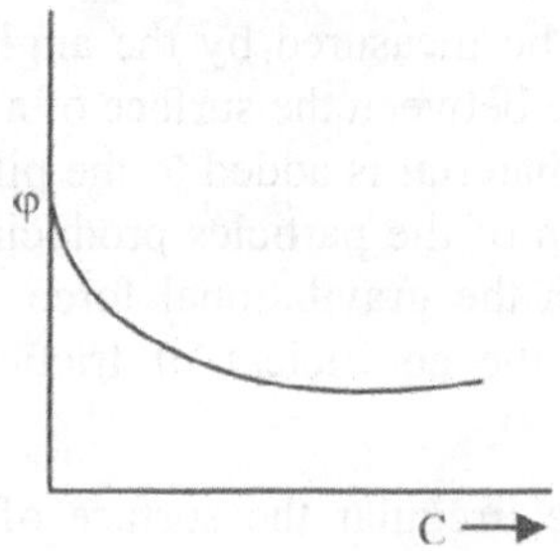

Fig. 29.1

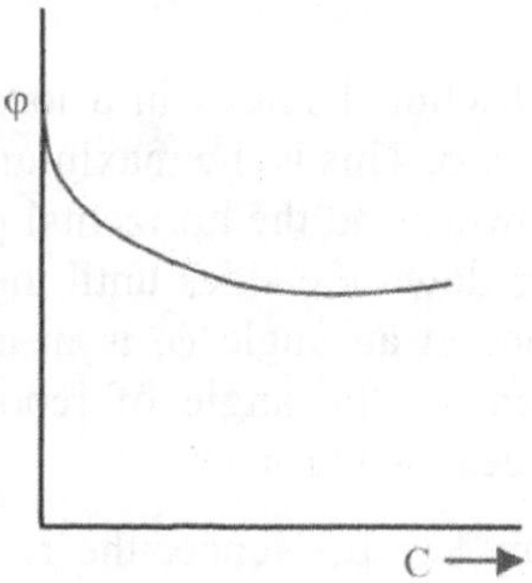

Fig. 29.2 Particle size (mm).

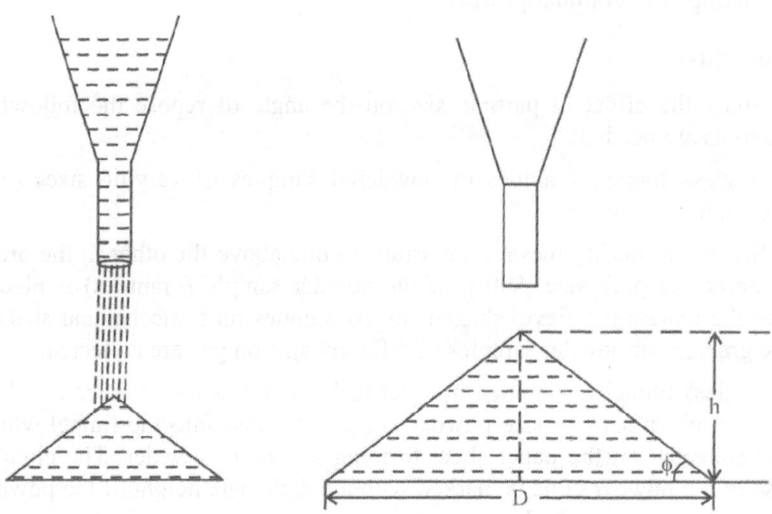

(a) Initial Stage (b) Final Stage

Fig. 29.3 Angle of repose determination by static funnal method.

$$\left(\text{Angle of Repose} = \phi = \tan^{-1}\frac{h}{r(0/2)}\right)$$

Precautions:

1. The funnel should not be fixed at a very high level from base,
2. The powder sample be added slowly through the funnel
3. The height of the cone "h" to be measured very carefully (one may use thin metal wire for the purpose)

Experiment – 29A

The Effect of Glidant Concentration on the Angle of Repose of a given Sample

A glass funnel, $CaCO_3$ powder (passed through a sieve mesh size and retained on the second sieve of a suitable combination), Magnesium stearate or Talc as glidants.

Procedure:

5 to 6 intimate mixture of the supplied sample (powder or granules) and the glidant are prepared as follows :

Table 29A.1

Mixture No.	1	2	3	4	5	6	7
Wt. of the powder (g)	25	24.8	24.6	24.4	24.0	23.5	23.0
Wt. of the glidant (g)	0	0.2	0.4	0.6	1.0	1.5	2.0
% glidant (w/w)	0	0.8	1.6	2.4	4.0	6.0	8.0
Or of any other suitable combinations							

The angle of repose for each mixture is then calculated (as already described in Experiment 29A). The height of the cone and its radius are also determined in each case. The observations are arranged in Tabular Form

Table 29A.2

Mixture No	1	2	3	4	5	6	7
% glidant	0.0	0.8	1.6	2.4	4.0	6.0	8.0
Radius, r (cm)							
Height, h (cm)							
$\tan \varphi = h/r$							
φ^o							

A graph is then plotted [φ *vs* cone of glidant (Figure 29A.3)]

Result: From the graph (Figure 29A.3) it is evident that as the concentration of the glidant is increased the angle of repose goes on decreasing indicating that "flowability" is increasing (over a limited range of glidant concentrations)

Experiment - 30

Determination of Swelling Index and Swelling Rate Constant of a Polymer

Swelling controlled release systems have a widespread application in pharmaceutical field. The water uptake by polymeric system generally termed as swelling. In the literature these systems are identified by different terms, like swelling controlled release system, hydrogel matrices or polymeric matrices exhibiting moving boundaries. In hydrogels of certain compositions, water can bind with the polymer chains, creating a rigid area around the mesh that is not accessible to solute or solvent diffusion. This can influence the transport of drug from the system.

Water uptake and drug delivery from swelling controlled release system can be described sufficiently by two dimensionless parameters. The diffusional Deborah number, De, which relates water motion to the rate of polymer relaxation.

$$De = \lambda/\varphi = (\lambda D_{1,2})/[\delta(t)]^2$$

λ = the characteristic relaxation time for the polymer when subjected to swelling stresses θ is the characteristic penetrant diffusion time into a swelling.

The swelling interface number, S_w is important in describing the balance between solvent penetration and solute diffusion.

$S_w = \nu\ \delta r/D_{3,2,1}$ [ν = velocity of the moving glasses)

δ = thickness of polymer.

$D_{3,2}$ is the diffusion coefficient of solute in the polymer)

The Swelling Index (S.I.) is calculated as :

$$S.I = \frac{\text{Final wt of the swollen polymer} - \text{wt of dry polymer}}{\text{weight of dry polymer}} \times 100$$

Process:

Accurately weighed 100 mg of polymer (Poly acrylic acid) is placed in muslin bag and tied. This bag is immersed in water and kept for several hours. Two hour interval the polymer was taken out and surface was dried by soaking the excess water with the help of a filter paper and weighed when two constant weight were obtained that was considered as equilibrium swelling and swelling Index was calculated as per equation-1.

Table 30.1 Weight of dry polymer = X_o (100 mg)

Time	Weight of swelling polymer
t_1	X_1
t_2	X_2
--	--
--	--
t_{n-1}	X_n
t_n	X_n

Swelling Index (S.I.) = $(X_n - X_o)/X_o \times 100\%$

Experiment - 31

Tablet Coating Procedures

The following instructions in routine sugar coating of tablets may be used as guide in the development of techniques for the coating of tablets in conventional coating equipment:

Formulas for the several component layers of the coating are offered for the purpose of permitting the students to vary these procedures in evolving better technique

Experiment - 31A

Sub-coating

Sub-coating Liquids:

Formula-1: Gelatin, granular = 2 ounces
Granulated sugar = 1½ pounds
Water = 1 pint

The gelatin is sprinkled onto the surface of the pint of cold water contained in the top of a double boiler, stirred until the gelatin is thoroughly distributed. The container with the prepared mixture is placed into the bottom of the double boiler which has been previously set to boiling, heated until the gelatin dissolves and then sugar is added and stirred until dissolved.

This solution is kept at 50°C when coating is being done. It congeals at room temperature when removing a dipperful for coating, the scum that forms on the surface must be pushed aside first.

The solution should be freshly prepared before use. Any unused potion should be discarded at the end of the day. The solution must not be over heated at any time. Maximum temperature should not exceed 70°C.

Formula-2: Gelatin, granular = 1 lb, 3 ounces
Granulated sugar = 15 lbs
Acacia, powdered = 1 lb
Water = 1 ½ gallon

Formula-3: Acacia, powdered = 1 lb
Corn Syrup = 1 lb
Syrup, I.P./U.S.P. = 1 gal.

Sub-coating Powders:

Formula-1: Calcium carbonate, Ppt = 4 part
Corn Starch = 1 part
Talc = 1 part

Mixed and passed through comminutor at high speed with fine screen and impacted forward.

Formula-2:	Kaolin	=	10 ½ ounces
	Calcium Carbonate	=	4 ½ ounces
	Powdered Sugar	=	2 ½ ounces
	Talc	=	3 ounces
	Terra Alba	=	2 ounces
	Acacia, Powdered	=	0 ½ ounce
Formula-3:	Powdered Sugar	=	14 ounces
	Powdered Acacia	=	2 ounces

Procedure:

1. 10 pounds of 'Terra Alba Placebo Tablets' are screened to remove all loose powder, granules, or broken tablets.
2. The coating pan is then loaded. The pan is not to be rotated until ready for coating. A steady blast of hot air is applied to pre-warm the tablets. This prevents the hot sub-coating liquid from congealing too quickly when applied.
3. When tablets are warm the hot air supply is shut off and the pan motor is started.
4. A sufficient quantity of the hot sub-coating liquid in a thin stream is applied over the rotating tablets until they are uniformly wetted. After this operation, manual stirring of the tablets is started immediately, removing a handful of them from time to time, to examine and see if all the tablet faces and edges are wet. If not, more of the liquid is added and the tablets are stirred again.

   NOTE: It is important that all the tablet edges be wetted; otherwise the subsequent applications of dusting powder will not adhere to the edges and this will result in a concavity at the edges.

   If too much liquid is added, the tablets will stop rolling and begin to stride. Should this occur, manual stirring will needed until they begin to roll again.

   [Hot Air on the Wet Tablets should be used at any time]
5. The amount of the liquid which was used is to be noted as a guide for later applications.
6. The tablets are then permitted to roll again until they become tacky and start to clump together.
7. At this point, a quantity of dusting powder is applied, stirred and then examined by removing a handful of tablets. If not spots are still visible, more powder is added until the tablets seem to be covered with a rather heavy layer of dry powder

[The beginner is cautioned against using too little or too much powder at this point. If an insufficient amount is used, the coating will either build up too slowly or else result in a rough coating. If too much powder is used, the excess amount not getting adsorbed by the wet tablets will collect in the rear of the coating pan. If this is not removed, the air blasts which are applied to dry the coating will blow the powder out into the room or subsequent applications of the hot sub-coating liquid will form little granules with the loose powders which will attach themselves to the coating causing the formation of very uneven tablets.]

8. When sufficient powder has been added, the tablets are allowed to roll for about five minutes and then hot air is applied. This is necessary to drive off the moisture in the coating and "set" it before proceeding to the next coating.

   [Hot air supply is not to be applied until this point or else it may drive off the powder before the tablets can adsorb a sufficient quantity. However, it is very important to drive off all moisture before applying the next coating or else the moisture may get sealed into the tablet or the coating can cause trouble in the later stage.

9. The tablets are allowed to roll under the hot air for at least 15 minutes or until the coating has hardened sufficiently to resist being peeled away from the tablet when the thumbnail is scrapped across coating.

10. After becoming certain that the tablets are quite dry, the hot air is shut off and steps 4 to 9 are repeated again.

    [Additional Notes] :

    (a) Should you observe excess powder in the rear of the pan, it should be removed with a small scoop before proceeding with the next coating.

    (b) During the early stages of sub-coating, some tablets may cling together and form "twins" or "triplets". These are generally observed rolling toward the front of the pan. These clusters are to be removed. Do not pull them apart and allow them to return to the pan.

    (c) Generally, at least 6 such coatings are required before the edges of the tablets are successfully rounded. At times, as many as 10 or 12 coats are needed. However, the fewer the number of coats that are used to produce a rounded edge, the less danger of producing a rough coating which will required many applications of smoothing coats later.

    (d) A record of the approximate volume of sub-coating liquid used is to be maintained together with the amounts of sub-coating powder. A good idea is to weigh 10 tablets before sub-coating, then weigh 10 more again after the sub-coating has been completed and the tablets are thoroughly dried. This will act as a guide for future coating projects. (Use Tablet Coating Control Sheet for this purpose).

(e) Finally; take your time! Do not attempt to rush the job as this will only result in expending more energy and time in the final stages of the coating procedure. Resist the urge to apply another coating before the previous one has been thoroughly dried.

Experiment - 31B

Sub-Coating

In order to reduce the time and effort involved in producing a uniform and satisfactory color coating it is essential that the sub-coating be made as smooth as possible. Very often, even the experienced coater produces a sub-coating which is pitted and covered with bumps and hollows. The smoothing coat serves to fill in the hollows and cover, or reduce, the bumps. The number of smoothing coats required will vary from batch to batch, depending on how well the sub-coating had been applied.

Smoothing Syrups:

Formula 1:	Granular Sugar	=	2 lbs
	Water	=	1 pint (= 473 mL)

1 pint (= 473 mL) is heated almost to boiling, then the sugar is added with stirring until it had dissolved. Heating is continued until the syrup begins to boil. It is allowed to boil for 2 to 3 minutes more with continuous stirring. If necessary, the hot syrup is strained through cheese cloth or muslin and the syrup temperature is maintained at a temperature between 60 to 65°C. This concentration of sugar will crystallize if permitted to cool.

Formula 2:	Calcium Carbonate	=	2 lbs
	Magnesium Carbonate	=	1 ½ lbs
	Powdered Sugar	=	4 lbs
	Methyl paraben	=	2 grams
	Water	=	1 gallon

The insoluble powders are blended into the water with continuous stirring until a smooth paste is obtained. It is heated to 60°C and the sugar is added with stirring until dissolved. It is then passed through colloid mill, if necessary, to produce a smooth, uniform suspension.

This suspension may be used when warm or at room temperature. It should be agitated before use.

Formula 3:	Calcium Carbonate	=	19% (w/w)
	Tricalcium Phosphate	=	1.0% (w/w)
	Syrup, U.S.P.	=	80% (w/w)

Formula 4: Powdered Sugar = 6 labs
Syrup, U.S.P. = 1 gallon

Choice of the smoothing syrup formula depends on several factors : (a) smoothness of sub-coating (b) size of the base (c) availability of equipment for either manufacturing the syrup or maintaining it at proper temperature and (d) experience of operator.

Generally, the concentrated clear syrup are useful for smooth routine operations. The suspensions (Formulas 2 & 3) are recommended for rapid building of rather rough sub-coatings.

Procedure:

1. One application of U.S.P. syrup is applied directly over the sub-coating. A sufficient volume of syrup is used to just wet the tablets, then hot air is applied for drying.
2. A quantity of the smoothing syrup is then applied in the same manner as described for sub-coating. The tablets are stirred manually, a handful of them is removed for inspection to see if the edges are all uniformly wet. In this, as well as, in subsequent coats, care, must be taken in the step of adding not too little or too much syrup. Too much syrup may result in producing tablets that would have adsorbed mixture which will be trapped as the coating dries and hardness.
3. The tablets are allowed to roll until they are almost dry and the coating becomes dull in appearance. At this point, the hot air is allowed to run in and the process continued to dry the tablets until the coating is hard.
4. Once the tablets are thoroughly dry and hard rolling of the tablets in the coating pan is discontinued. Otherwise, the coating may get chipped or cracked.
5. The smoothing syrup application operation may be continued in this fashion till the tablets are smooth and the obvious pits and bumps are removed.

   [*Note:* If the sub-coating is very rough, applying several coats may be tried in the same manner as described above, but the mouth of the pan should be covered with plastic sheeting after each application of syrup. This delays evaporation and permits the syrup to soften and smooth the very large bumps]

   It needs to be emphasized that a good color coating depends on a very smooth and hard base coating for uniformity of color deposition. After successful removal of the gross hollows and bumps from the sub-coating the next step involves laying down an even smoother base for the colored syrup. This may be accomplished as follows:

6. The coating pan is required to be made clean and dry; the tablets are not permitted to roll when dry. This is a must from this point onward.

   U.S.P. syrup is to be used. Just enough syrup is applied to the tumbling tablets to wet the faces and edges. Stirring is done manually to permit the tablets to roll until they become dull in appearance. Then cool air is turned on and the tablets are allowed to dry up.

   It is observed that drying syrup coatings in this manner is much quicker than previous coats. Generally, only about 4 to 5 minutes are required to dry the coating. If the smoothing coating procedure has been carefully carried out only about 3 to 5 such coatings are required. The tablets at this point should be very smooth in appearance when examined with a hand lens of 10 to 14 power.

Experiment - 31C

Coloring

The classic procedures in pan color coating involve the careful and tedious procedure of slowly building up the color onto the tablets by starting with dilute solutions of dyes in syrup and gradually increasing the concentration of dye in the syrup. This procedure often requires the application of from 150 to 250 separate coats in order to achieve the desired shade and uniformity of color deposition. This method is advantageous in that it rarely produces mottled or spotted color coats. It obvious disadvantage is the expenditure of time involved.

Procedure (A): (3 days' programme)

1. An aqueous concentrate of a suitable FD&C color is prepared. It is suggested that light pastel shades be used for the first attempt at coloring. The solution is prepared by dissolving 1.0g of the color in sufficient water to make 100 mL of solution. This 1% (w/w) solution should be stored in battle, suitably labeled.
2. To 5 mL of the color concentrate U.S.P. syrup is added to make it a 250 mL volume, stirred well until thoroughly mixed and this syrup is applied as before. In applying the syrup a small graduate is used to measure up the volume which is required to just wet the tablets uniformly. The exact same volume is then used for all subsequent coats until it becomes apparent that this volume no longer is sufficient to thoroughly wet the tablets as they increase in bulk and cost. When this occurs, increased volume of syrup is tried.
3. If a light shade of the color is desired, the ratio of 5 mL of the concentrate to 250 mL of the syrup is used in operations until the tablets are uniformly colored. However, if a deeper shade is desired, the amount of the concentrate is increased to 10 mL, then 15 mL, or higher as each 250 mL portion of colored syrup is exhausted and a fresh batch is required to be prepared. One means of judging the color of the finished tablet is to follow the rule that the color of the finished tablet will be slightly deeper than the color of the syrup being used. This may vary with different colors, however.

   [*Note*: Hot air blasts are to be used only during the final stages of drying each application. The interior of the coating pan is not permitted to become rough as the color coating operation proceeds. If necessary, the tablets are to be removed and the pan is thoroughly washed, cleared and dried].

Procedure (B): (- 6 – 8 hours)

An accelerated alternative procedure of depositing color coats reduces the number of individual applications to 16 to 20 coats. This method requires extremely smooth tablets to begin with an a certain degree of experience in pan coating.

1. 36° Baume Syrup is prepared by bringing one gallon of water to boiling and then adding 22 pounds of granulated sugar. Heat is continued with stirring until all the sugar is dissoloved, then added 4g of Methyl Paraben and 2 grams if Propyl Paraben which will get dissolved in hot syrup.

   This solution must be kept hot. Therefore, the syrup is prepared in a steam-jacketed stainless steel kettle and maintained at 35-40°C. The concentration of the syrup should be checked at intervals with a Baume Hydrometer and additional water is added when required to maintain the desired concentration of sugar in solution.

   This solution may be kept from one working day to the next by simply reheating the re-crystallized syrup the following day. This concentration should always be checked following reheating and adjusted to 36°B.

2. *Preparation of color stock solution:* The concentration of this solution will vary from 1 – 4% depending on solubility of the component dyes in water and the color desired on the finished tablets.

   For laboratory size batches of 10 points of tablets, 100 mL of Color Stock Solution is usually adequate. It is prepared as follows:
   (a) 20 mL of water is heated to boil.
   (b) The required chosen dye is then added and heating continued till it is dissolved.
   (c) Heat source is removed, and the syrup concentrate (36°B) is added to bring the volume to 100 mL.

3. The accelerated color coating technique involves adding highly-colored hot, concentrated syrup in increasing increments of 10% until uniformly colored tablets are obtained. This is accomplished by diluting portions of the Color Stock Solution with 36°B Syrup and applying two coats of each of these dilutions at 10, 20, 30, 40 and 50% levels.

At this point, the tablets are generally uniformly colored. If they are not, then 2 applications of each successive dilution of 60, 70, 80 and 90% levels are added.

4. When the tablets are uniformly covered, the intensity of the color is adjusted by adding the color stock solution directly for at least 2 to 6 coats.
5. Hot or warm air may be used to completely dry each application. The tablets are not permitted to roll for any considerable length of time after they have been dried.

   [*Note*: Record the exact volumes of each application and be sure that you use enough to just adequate cover the tablets each time. A graduate may be used to measure exact volumes when applying syrup].
6. When the color-coating has been completed, a finishing coating of 32°B uncolored syrup is applied as follows: (Do not use air blasts).

   Just enough of the 32^{0}B syrup is applied to cover the tablets uniformly. The amount used here should be that amount which had been used by means of a graduate during the earlier stages just prior to the finishing operation.

   The tablets are stirred and observed carefully. Just as soon as they become dull in appearance, a volume of uncolored syrup equal to $3/4^{th}$ of the volume of the first application is applied. Manual stirring is done again and the rotating tablets observed closely. As soon as they again become dull in appearance, a volume of uncolored syrup equal to ½ the volume of the first application is added again.

   Stirring process is repeated followed by close watching. Just as soon as the tablets' appearance begin to become dull, the motor is shut off and the coating pan is stopped. The pan is then immediately covered with a plastic or canvas sheet ensuring tight covering.
7. Every 5 minutes thereafter, the coating pan is rotated for ¼ of turn by flipping the switch on and off as quickly as possible. The pan must not be permitted to make a complete revolution as far as practicable. The pan is to be rotated in this manner for 30 to 45 minutes. The cover is not to be removed to look at the tablets.
8. At the end of this period the tablets should have dried to dull but very smooth finish. The motor is started again and tablets are rotated for about 5-6 minutes to insure complete dryness.

   The over all length of time required for final drying intervals will vary with atmospheric conditions in the coating room. In rooms without controlled humidity, it may be wiser to extend these time limitations under conditions of high humidity.

Polishing:

The final stage in the coating process consists of polishing the coated tablets to achieve a high luster. There are several methods (currently employed) to polish tablets as well as many formulas for the polishing solution. A special canvas-lined pan or drum is employed during this stage.

The polishing operation should be carried on in a dust free atmosphere. This means that attempts should not be made to polish tablets in the same coating room with another operator applying sub-coating powder to his batch of tablets.

Since, many of the solution solvents used in the solution of waxes are flammable, be sure that no open flames are there, anywhere in the room. Also the fumes that are thrown off from the polishing pan during and after the solution is applied it must not be inhaled.

Polishing Solutions

Formula 1:	White Beeswax	=	15 g
	High Grade Carnauba Wax	=	10 g
	Chloroform	=	500 mL.

In preparing the polishing solution, the solvent is made to get warmed in one container and the waxes are allowed to melt in another. Then, the solvent is carefully added to the fused waxes and heating is continued until a clear solution results.

Formula 2:	Bareco, 190 (Microcrystalline wax)	=	15% (w/v)
	Tween 80	=	3 or 4% (w/v)
	Carbon Tetrachloride	=	q.s. 100%
Formula 3:	Bareco 190 wax	=	50%
	Carnauba wax	=	50%
Formula-4:	Carnauba wax	=	3 parts
	Paraffin	=	2 parts
	White Beeswax	=	2 parts

Formulas 3 and 4 are polishing waxes applied dry to the tablets or used to first line the interior of the polishing pan by flowing the fused mass into the pan and allowing it to congeal. The tablets are then added to the pan and rotated till they acquire a high polish.

Procedure:

1. The dry tablets are transferred to the polishing pan. Just prior to adding the polishing the motor is to be started.

2. The polishing solution should be added while it is just warm enough to maintain solution of the waxes, but never while it is HOT! 100 mL is generally sufficient for a batch of 50,000 tablets.

   Formula 1 is used for a 10 lb batch of tablets by diluting 10 mL of the warm solution with 5 mL. of chloroform ($CHCl_3$) for the first application.

3. The motor is started, the solution is poured onto the tablets in a thin stream while stirring them manually.

   [*Note:* Be sure your hand is DRY: DO NOT USE AIR BLASTS AT ANY TIME DURING THE POLISHING OPERATION]

The tablets are allowed to roll for 10 minutes, then is added a 5 mL. portion of undiluted Formula-1. A second application is recommended for polishing the tablets for an additional 20-30 minutes.

[***Remember:*** You can always add more of the solution if required – but you can ruin the finish of the tablets by adding too much at once. Watch the tablets for about 20 minutes. They should show signs of a polish by then. If not, another 5 mL. of the polishing solution may be allowed and the tablets allowed to roll until they acquire a high shine.

Note: Do not try to 'improve' on the shine of the tablets by permitting them to roll for an extended period after they have been satisfactorily polished. This may result in chipped or cracked coatings]

Experiment - 32

Evaluation of Tablets

Tablets are usually required to be tested for the following

Characteristics

1. ***General appearance:*** The general appearance of a tablet allows monitoring lot-to-lot or tablet-to-tablet uniformity in terms of size, shape, surface, smoothness, shine, etc.
2. ***Hardness and friability:*** Tablet hardness affects both tablet disintegration and drug dissolution. If these tablets are too hard, it may not disintegrate within the required period or meet the dissolution specification. If they are too soft, they will not withstand the handling and shipping operations. Certain tablets that are intended to dissolve slowly (e.g. sustained-release tablets) are made hard. Other tablets that are intended to dissolve rapidly (and for quick onset of drug action) are made soft. Friability is the tendency of the tablets to crumble.
3. ***Weight and content uniformity:*** 20 tablets are usually weighed individually and the average weight is calculated to ensure that the contain the desired amounts of drug substances, with little variation among contents within a tablet.
4. ***Disintegration:*** Disintegration of tablets is evaluated to ensure that the drug substance is fully available for dissolution and absorption from the GI Tract. A maximum time for disintegration to occur is specified for each type of tablet. The disintegration media requires vary depending on the type of tablets to be tested according to U.S.P. specifications. The disintegration test is used as a control for tablets intended to be administered by mouth, but not for the chewable and sustained release types.
5. ***Dissolution:*** Because drug abs option and physiological availability depend on having the drug agent in the dissolved state, suitable dissolution characteristics are important properties of tablets. The dissolution test provides a means of control to ensure that a given formulating is the same with regard to dissolution as the batch of tablets shown initially to be clinically effective.

Experiment - 33

Thermodynamics of Solubilization (i.e. Micellar Solubilization)

Miceller solubilization may be considered as a partitioning of the drug between the micellar phase and the aqueous environment. Thus, the standard Gibbs' Free Energy change of solubilization, ΔG^{o} can be computed from the partition coefficient, K, determination of the miceller/aq. Medium.

$$K = \frac{C_{micelle}}{C_{aq.medium}} \text{ \& the required eqn. for } \Delta G^{o} = (-\, RT \text{ in } K) \qquad .....(1)$$

where, K has the usual significance of partition coefficient between the micellar phase and aqueous environment.

The standard free enthalpy change (ΔH^{o}) and entropy change (ΔS^{o}) of solubilization can be computed from the usual relationships.

$$\ln K = \frac{\Delta H_{S}^{o}}{RJ} + \text{Constant} \qquad .....(2)$$

$$\text{Log } K_2/K_1 = \frac{-\,\Delta H_{S}^{0}[1/T_2 - 1/T_1]}{2.303\text{ R}} = \frac{+\,\Delta H_{s}^{o}}{2.303\text{ R}}\left(\frac{T_2 - T_1}{T_1 T_2}\right) \qquad .....(3)$$

R = universal gas constant and

T = the temp. of the experimental set up in Kalvin scale.

$$\text{And } \Delta G_{s}^{o} = \Delta H_{s} - T\Delta S_{s} \qquad .....(4)$$

When ΔG_s is positive (i.e. $\Delta G_{s}^{o} > 0$) solubilization will not occur. When ΔS_{s}^{o} calculated is positive, more disordered is the system and the reverse will be the case when $\Delta S_s < 0$ i.e. positive. The thermodynamic functions ΔH^{o} and ΔS^{o} are due to several kinds of interactions. Donor-acceptor and H-bonding are associated with both negative ΔH^{o} and $-\ \Delta S^{o}$, the large negative ΔH^{o} values overcoming the unfavorable entropy chage. Thus ΔG_{S}^{o}, if negative, the solubilization process is spontaneous.

Procedure:

1. A weighed amount (accurately known) of the experimental material is added to a known volume of the aqueous medium (if required, in a buffered solvent of desired pH.) and shaken (or stirred) for some time.
2. A measured quantity (in volume terms) of the surfactant solution of known HLB value is then added drop-wise from the burette (or graduated pipette) while stirring it thoroughly until the critical micellar concentration (cmc) point is reached and slightly exceeded. The resulting system is stirred for a few more minutes.
3. The system is then allowed to stand undisturbed for some more time to allow the equilibrium to be achieved.
4. With the help of a graduated pipette a measured aliquot of the aqueous medium is withdrawn and assayed by a convenient and suitable analytical method.
5. The amount partitioned in the micellar phase is then calculated by subtracting the amount assayed from the aqueous phase from the total amount initially added.
6. The partition coefficient (or distribution coefficient) of the experimental substance, K, between the micellar and aqueous phases is then computed by using the equation:

   $$K = \frac{C_{micelle}}{C_{aq.\ medium}}$$

   Where, $C_{micellar} = W_1 - W_2$ (W_1 being the initial weight taken and W_2 is the weight as calculated taking the whole volume of the aqueous phases into consideration).

   [*Note:* While withdrawing the aliquot from the aqueous phase care should be taken so as to avoid drawing any micellar phase into the pipette. A teflon plug attached at the tip of the pipette will be of help in this matter. Withdrawal from the interface must be avoided as the concentration of the surfactant at the interface is more than that in the bulk of each phase].
7. The above experiment is repeated at another temperature so as to calculate the value of ΔH_s^o, the enthalpy change i.e. the latent heat involved in micellar solubilization by using the equation (3).

   Alternatively, the partition coefficient determination procedure is repeated at varying temperatures (prefixed) and computing K value for each temperature from the equation (1) a plot of logK vs 1/T may be drawn using equation (2) and from the resulting straight line plot slope value will be obtained. Then using the slope value, ΔH_s^o latent heat of micellar solubilization (i./e. enthalpy change) may be computed.

[Eqn. is Slope = $\frac{\Delta H_s^o}{2.303 \times R}$ jR = 1.987 Cal/(mol)(K)]

8. Then from the calculated values of ΔG_s and ΔH_s the entropy change, ΔS_s , involved in the process can be computed using the equation (4).

Experiment – 33A

Thermodynamics of Micellization

For a non-ionic surfactant, in a single-step to form a micelle, M, the equation is:

$$n\,S \rightleftharpoons M \text{ (micelle molecule)} \qquad \text{.....(1)}$$

and equilibrium constant

$$K_m = \frac{[M]}{[S]^n} \qquad \text{.....(2)}$$

When n = Number of surfactant molecules S that come together to form a single micelle M.

Conventional thermodynamic arguments then show that when n is large, then the free energy change, ΔG^o_m of micelle formation at the cmc is :

$$\Delta G^o_M = -RT\ \text{In}\ K_M = -RT\ \text{In}\ K_{CMC(M)} \qquad \text{.....(3)}$$

$$= -RT\ln\frac{[m]}{[S]_{CMC}} \text{ (for non-ionic surfactant)} \qquad \text{.....(4)}$$

Where ΔG^o_M represents the standard free-energy change for transferring 1 mole of S(SAA) from aqueous solution into its micelle.

In the formation of micelle (ionic, involving anionic or cationic) let us suppose n number of S ions together with m number of counter ions form a charged micelle (+ve / -ve) i.e. :

$$nS^{(-ve/+ve)} + m^{(+ve/-ve)} \rightleftharpoons M^{Q(-ve/+ve)}$$

where n = aggregation number and m = no. of counter ions bound to the micelle δQ = (n-m) and $\Delta G_M{}^0$ / n then becomes the standard free energy change per mole of surfactant monomer (molecule).

At the cmc condition, $\Delta G^o/M$ is finally given by the equation :

$$\Delta G^o_{mic} = RT\ln(CMC) + RT$$

$$= RT\,(1 + m/n)\ln(cmc)$$

$$= RT\left\{1 + \frac{(n - Q)}{n}\right\} \text{in (cmc)}$$

$$= RT\left\{2 - \frac{Q^{-ve/+ve}}{n}\right\} \text{in (cmc)}$$

Now, knowing the cmc value, the aggregation number n, and the net charge difference (+ve/–ve) on the micelle, $\Delta G^0{}_{mic}$ for an anionic or cationic micelle can be obtained

The charge difference can be measured by conductivity measurement and the equation applied is $\lambda_\infty = \pi_c/\pi_\infty$

For non-ionic surfactant, m = 0, the equation is then

$$\Delta G^o_{mic} = RT \ln (cmc)$$

The standard enthalpy and entropy changes of micallization can be computed from the expressions:

$$\ln (cmc) = \frac{-\Delta H^o_{mic} 1/T}{R} + \frac{\Delta S^o_{mic}}{R}$$

Or $$\log (cmc) = \frac{-\Delta H^o_{mic} 1/T}{2.303R} + \frac{\Delta S^o_{mic}}{2.303R}$$

$$\Delta G^o_{mic} = \Delta H^o_{mic} - T\Delta S^o_{mic}$$

By determining the cmc values of the surfactant system at varying temperature and plot graph of log(cmc) vs 1/T an Arrhenius plot-like graph (a straight line) will result from the slope of which

[Slope = ΔH^o_{mic} /(2.303)(R)] the enthalpy change can be computed and the intercept on the Y-axis will yield a value equal to ΔS^o_{mic} / (2.303)R from which the standard entropy change, ΔS^o_{mic} involved is obtained.

Thus, the thermodynamic functions become known to us for such a process. In fact, this is the approach for such process as mechanisms.

